T0367162

Miracle Cure

For Chris, Anna and Robert

Miracle Cure

*The Story of Penicillin and the
Golden Age Of Antibiotics*

Milton Wainwright

Basil Blackwell

Copyright © Milton Wainwright 1990

First published 1990

Basil Blackwell Ltd
108 Cowley Road, Oxford, OX4 1JF, UK

Basil Blackwell, Inc.
3 Cambridge Center
Cambridge, Massachusetts 02142, USA

British Library Cataloguing in Publication Data
A CIP catalogue record for this book is available from the British Library.

Library of Congress Cataloging in Publication Data
Wainwright, Milton.
Miracle cure: the story of antibiotics / Milton Wainwright.
p.   cm.
Includes bibliographical references.
ISBN 0–631–16492–8
1.   Antibiotics – History.   1.   Title.
[DNLM.   1.   Antibiotics – History.   QV 11.1 W142m]
RM267.W24   1990
615′.329′09–dc20
DNLM/DLC
for Library of Congress   89-17601
                                   CIP

Typeset in 11 on 12 pt Sabon
by Joshua Associates Ltd, Oxford

In 1958 Carl Dauer, of the US National Office of Vital Statistics, estimated that 1.5 million lives had been saved during the preceding 15 years as the result of the introduction of sulphonamides, penicillin and the other antibiotics.

Contents

Preface

This book provides an account of the discovery and development of antibiotics, a wide range of chemical substances produced by micro-organisms which have the ability to kill or inhibit pathogens and which have had a major impact on the treatment of infectious disease. No doubt because of the miraculous effect which the introduction of antibiotics had on medicine, their story is one of the most thoroughly researched and often related in medical history. Although penicillin, the first of the true antibiotics, was discovered some sixty years ago, its story continues to interest the general public and, amongst medical historians at least, generates some fierce debate.

The statistician can readily demonstrate that improvements in public health, nutrition and general medical practice had begun to make an impact on infectious diseases long before antibiotics appeared on the scene. While this is true, the newly discovered antibiotics had a major impact on medicine and on the public's imagination because of their ability to produce dramatic, last-minute cures of patients who had seemed certain to die. It seemed to the public that antibiotics were a wonder drug, a miracle cure.

In this book I have tried to give an uncomplicated account of the discovery of these compounds. Although aimed primarily at the general reader, I hope that the book will also be of interest to the microbiologist or medical specialist, who may be only vaguely familiar with the history of antibiotics. Throughout, I have avoided the use of technical terms or, where this was not possible, at least explained them. To the medically trained eye, this may occasionally make the prose seem simplistic; my main aim, however, has been to avoid too much specialized termino-logy, in the hope that the general reader will be able to share my interest in the many fascinating aspects of the story of antibiotics.

Rather than give a fully detailed academic account I have tried to select the most interesting aspects of the antibiotics story. Similarly, I have not provided detailed references to my source material, although a fairly comprehensive list of further reading material is provided. I realize that this approach may offend some academic medical historians, but I felt that footnotes and individual reference citations would ruin the narrative flow for the general reader. However, I would welcome correspondence from any reader who is particularly interested in the source of any information which I have referred to.

The opening chapters are devoted to the story of penicillin. In fact, the history of this one antibiotic makes up nearly half of the book. For this I make no apologies. The penicillin story is by far the most well researched in the history of antibiotics and is the one which most readily catches the public's imagination, so it clearly deserves as full a treatment as possible within the limitations of available space. There is much new information in these chapters. In particular I have discussed recent studies concerning the first confirmed use of penicillin. I have also attempted to redress recent attempts to downgrade the role played by Sir Alexander Fleming in the discovery of this the most famous antibiotic. I hope that by adopting this approach I have not correspondingly fallen into the trap of being unfair to the Oxford group, whose contribution to the development of penicillin was obviously of paramount importance.

In the chapter titled 'The Road to Antibiotics', I have provided a retrospective on the precursors of the antibiotics, including an account of the use of mould therapy in ancient as well as more recent folk medicine. Also included is a description of the even more bizarre use of live maggots to treat infections. This illustrates the extremes to which doctors were prepared to go to achieve a cure before they had ready access to antibiotics.

The history of streptomycin, the second major antibiotic to appear, is given in chapter 8. This is the first detailed account of this story to be published, and in it I have once again attempted to redress an historical imbalance, this time in favour of Albert Schatz, one of its co-discoverers. In doing so, I hope I have not been unfair to the memory of Selman Waksman, the co-discoverer who received all the credit for streptomycin.

The story of antibiotics such as chloramphenicol and nystatin, both products of the so-called 'golden age of antibiotics', is the topic to which chapter 9 is devoted. The last chapters are given over to a relatively short account of some recent developments which have taken place in the story of antibiotics. Here I have discussed the involvement of antibiotics in the treatment of medical problems such as cancer and viral infections like AIDS, which threatens to develop into one of the most devastating medical problems of all time. I end the book by speculating that antibiotics may one day be replaced by vaccines and, as a result, become as out of place in the medicine of the future as maggot therapy is today. The end of the antibiotics story is clearly a long way off, however. In the interim, we will continue to rely upon these compounds to defeat infections long known to humanity, and also perhaps to fight some of the newer diseases which have only recently become major problems. I hope that I have not concluded the book on a pessimistic note but, rather, have placed the story of antibiotics in the context of the history of medicine, the development of which has been typified by the continual introduction of new approaches to the fight against infection.

I would particularly like to thank Dr C. G. Paine and Professor R. J. V. Pulvertaft who kindly related accounts of their pioneering work with crude penicillin. I also had the privilege of interviewing Professor Albert Schatz concerning his role in the discovery of streptomycin. I am also grateful to him for the provision of much new archival material on this subject. I also wish to express my gratitude to Dr Hubert Lechevalier and the other members of staff of the Waksman Institute and Waksman Archive at Rutgers. Thanks also go to Professor Seymour Hutner of Pace University, New York; Mrs Brenda Ward for her account of the Twomey story; Lady Florey for allowing me to quote from her husband's letters; and to Dr Harold Swan, with whom I collaborated during research which led to the discovery of records of the first clinical use of penicillin. Finally I would like to thank Ms A. Lewis Clark for typing the first draft, Alan Hancock for expert photographic help, and Martin Hancock and Rowland Leathers for their introduction to the finer points of word processing. David Trott and John Cross of the Microbiology Department at Sheffield are also thanked for much miscellaneous, but nevertheless important help.

Financial assistance from the Wellcome Trust and Waksman Foundation is also gratefully acknowledged.

1

Introduction

London enjoyed splendid weather during the first few weeks of September 1928, with temperatures reaching the high seventies and then toppling over into the low eighties Fahrenheit. The autumn of that year had seen an alarming spread in Dutch elm disease throughout southern Britain, while more worrying events were being witnessed in other parts of the world. In Europe, arguments continued over the fate of the Rhinelands. In China a war raged. Nature, too, showed itself in a particularly vindictive mood, when a massive hurricane devastated Florida and the Caribbean, killing at least 800 people. The citizens of New South Wales, Australia, were more fortunate, having only a referendum on prohibition to worry about.

Although many of that autumn's events were tragic, or were to prove important to the future welfare of mankind, they were to be eclipsed by a discovery which failed to be reported even in the minor columns of the world's newspapers.

At the end of July 1928, the eminent Scottish bacteriologist, Alexander Fleming, left his laboratory at St Mary's Hospital, Paddington, in London, to spend the summer with his family at their cottage in Suffolk. As he closed the door on his laboratory, he was unaware that fate had already set in motion events which were to lead him to make perhaps the most important discovery in medicine. Fleming made an unscheduled return to his laboratory in September. Casually, he glanced at some petri dishes which he had inoculated with bacteria before going away on holiday. One of these dishes caught his eye, and at that moment penicillin was born. It would be another 12 years, however, before Howard Florey, Ernst Chain and a team of scientists at Oxford University would purify penicillin and give the world its first true antibiotic. From that point on the search for new, life-saving antibiotics began, and the antibiotic age was in full swing.

In 1978, some 50 years after Fleming's original discovery of penicillin, 12 million kilos of antibiotics were produced in the USA alone. Their impact on medicine can be gauged by the fact that, in the first 10 years after antibiotics became widely available, they had cut the death rate from 8 diseases which they influenced by over 50 per cent, saving some 80,000 lives. It is hardly surprising, then, that penicillin and the later antibiotics caught the public's imagination, and that Fleming and the other pioneers of the antibiotic age were honoured and fêted wherever they went.

It is difficult for those of us younger than 45, who are children of the antibiotic era, to fully appreciate the impact which the appearance of the antibiotics had on medicine. While it is true that by the late 1930s sulphonamides had already had a major influence on the treatment of bacterial infections, they were to prove far from ideal, largely because of the speed with which bacteria developed resistance to them. Most hospitals still had a septic ward which stank of the products of bacterial infection. It was possible to die from the most trivial examples of bacterial contamination, for example, after pricking one's finger on a thorn while gardening!

Penicillin's arrival was to change all that. It would also play a major role in the Allied victory in the Second World War. While the Axis powers were largely dependent upon the vagaries of sulphonamides, Allied troops stormed the beaches of Normandy in the knowledge that they were largely immune to the age-old battle diseases such as gangrene, pneumonia and septicaemia.

Soon after the War, a black market in penicillin developed throughout occupied Europe, providing rich pickings for the Mafia, and an unusual sub-plot for Graham Greene's novel, *The Third Man*. In fact, so desperate were the Germans for penicillin that they even imported large quantities of the urine of treated patients, from which they extracted the life-saving drug!

The impact of penicillin and the antibiotics which followed can be readily shown by the use of statistics, but it is perhaps best illustrated by accounts, some highly emotional, about the impact of these drugs on the lives of individual patients. A good example of such an account was recently given by Louise Carter, a Queen's nurse and retired midwife. In an article in *Nursing Mirror*, she describes how she first saw penicillin used in 1943 to treat a woman who was close to death, suffering from puerperal or childbed fever. The patient, a Mrs Phyllis Andrews, had given birth to a healthy baby but had contracted a bacterial infection of the womb which had spread throughout her system and was now threatening her life. Nurse Carter recalls how one evening she heard hurried footsteps outside her ward, and the consultant, a Mr Verwood, entered, already gowned and masked and obviously ready for action. He asked her for a 10 cc syringe of water and then began to scrub up. Taking the syringe, he injected the contents into one of two vials containing a yellow powder. The powder dissolved and immediately gave off a pungent smell, which somewhat shocked Nurse Carter. The solution was then injected into a bottle of dextrosesaline which was given as a drip into the woman's vein. Incredibly, after only half an hour the patient's blood pressure had begun to rise, her temperature had dropped two degrees, and her pulse had fallen to a reasonable level of ninety. The second bottle of the new drug was then given and by 5. 40 in the morning, Mrs Andrews opened her eyes and with some bewilderment asked for a cup of tea. Nurse Carter summed up her account in the following words: 'And so I left that happy little family, a proud relieved father, a beautiful contented baby and a happy young mother snatched from the very brink of death by a miracle drug.'

It is not surprising that penicillin had such an amazing impact on the doctors and nurses who first witnessed such dramatic effects. It seemed to be a new wonder drug, and at first it was used with almost complete abandon. Doctors began to prescribe it for all manner of infections, such as the common cold, against which it was totally ineffective. The misuse could not last forever, and the rapid appearance of penicillin-resistant bacteria almost reduced penicillin's 'wonder drug' status to the shortest on record. Worse was to follow, when penicillin-related deaths began to be reported. Fortunately, penicillin weathered these storms, and together with the antibiotics which followed, it completely changed the course of medical science.

Until relatively recently, it seemed as if the advent of the antibiotics and other major developments in medicine had finally conquered infectious disease. Then a whole series of new medical problems appeared or reasserted themselves: hepatitis B, genital herpes, antibiotic-resistant meningitis bacteria, salmonellosis, and most recently AIDS – all arose to challenge our cosy medical status quo. Fortunately, antibiotics continue to play a major role in combating both the traditional microbial infections, and also these newer manifestations, and the continued development of new compounds and new approaches to the use of established antibiotics promises to keep us ahead in our long-standing battle against infectious disease.

MICROORGANISMS AND DISEASE

The science of microbiology was a mere 50 years old by 1928, when Fleming first observed the penicillin phenomenon, yet remarkable progress had already been made in the study of bacteria, fungi, viruses and protozoa, many of which have the ability to cause devastating diseases such as cholera, histoplasmosis and poliomyelitis. Progress had also been made in the use of antiseptics and the development of effective means of treating sewage, developments which, when coupled with an overall improvement in public hygiene, were to have a major impact on the natural history of infectious disease.

It was soon found that bacteria were the cause of by far the majority of common infectious diseases. These minute, usually rod-shaped organisms are about three millionths of a metre (3μ) in diameter and produce a characteristically mucoid colony when growing on a nutrient agar. Although many bacteria are pathogens and cause disease in humans, most are saprophytes, which live by decomposing dead organic matter. As saprophytes, bacteria contribute to the cycling of nutrients, a process which is essential for life on earth. The list of human diseases caused by bacteria is a long one, and includes septicaemia, tetanus, anthrax, bacterial endocarditis, scarlet fever, diphtheria, pneumonia, tuberculosis, whooping cough, gonorrhea, septic meningitis, plague and indolent fever.

One group of bacteria, the actinomycetes, are also responsible for most of the antibiotics in current use. Of particular importance in this respect are the *Streptomyces*, filamentous organisms which, like all actinomycetes, were once regarded as fungi, but which for good reasons are now classed as bacteria. *Streptomyces* are the source of important antibiotics such as streptomycin, neomycin and nystatin.

In 1884, the Danish bacteriologist, Christian Gram, divided bacteria into two groups on the basis of their reaction to a stain which bears his name. The distinction between Gram-positive and Gram-negative bacteria is still widely used today to characterize bacteria. As we shall see, this distinction is important because some antibiotics act solely on either Gram positive or Gram negative bacteria, while some have a wide spectrum of activity and inhibit representatives of both groups.

Unlike the majority of bacteria, fungi are typically filamentous microorganisms, although the yeasts produce characteristic spherical cells which reproduce by budding. Fungi, or moulds as they are often called, are generally regarded as decomposer organisms, although they are extremely important plant pathogens. Less frequently, this group of microorganisms can cause disease in humans. Examples include somewhat trivial infections like athlete's foot and ringworm, more serious infections such as oral and vaginal thrush, and lastly life-threatening diseases like histoplasmosis. Some fungi, like many actinomycetes, also produce important antibiotics.

By far the majority of the microbial infections which are of particular worry today are caused by viruses, largely because we have no antibiotics and only a few drugs with which we can combat these remarkable infective agents. Viruses are extremely small and can be seen only with the aid of an electron microscope. They are approximately a thousandth of the volume of bacteria and, unlike most other microorganisms, cannot be cultivated on laboratory media, but must be grown either in tissue culture or on their hosts. Viruses cause diseases such as smallpox, chickenpox, herpes, rubella, mumps, yellow and Lassa fevers, influenza, the common cold and AIDS.

Protozoa provide the last major group of microorganisms. The vast majority of these are harmless, although some species cause major diseases like malaria, sleeping sickness and a form of dysentery.

For those readers who are not familiar with the techniques used by the microbiologist, it might prove useful for me to briefly discuss how microorganisms are grown and studied in the laboratory. Microorganisms exist all around us, in the air we breathe, on our skin and clothing and in the food we eat. As a result, the founding fathers of the science of microbiology had to develop methods of 'sterile technique', to ensure that they could isolate and work with individual microorganisms, rather than a mixed culture. The most essential requirement of this technique is that everything which the microbiologist uses to grow microbes must first be sterilized, generally in an autoclave (a machine which is essentially a large pressure cooker in which contaminating microorganisms are killed by a combination of heat and high pressure). The sterilized growth media can then be aseptically inoculated with spores or cells of individual microorganisms which are then grown and can be studied further. The growth media employed vary with the organism used. They may be liquid broths (not unlike gravy) or liquids containing essential nutrients in a more defined chemical form. Microorganisms are also conveniently grown on media solidified by the addition of agar. In this case, the agar medium is usually poured into glass or, more commonly nowadays, plastic petri dishes, in which it solidifies to form what is referred to as a 'plate'. The inoculated liquid media or plates are than incubated at a temperature which is optimal for the growth of the organism. Pathogenic bacteria are often cultivated on nutrient or meat broths or on solid media like blood agar. They are usually incubated at 37°C, at which temperature they generally grow overnight. Fungi are usually grown on media like the one first described by Czapek and Dox which bears their name. This medium contains all the nutrients essential for fungal growth, but not complex additives such as meat and yeast extract. It is referred to as a 'defined medium' in contrast to various 'undefined' media, the exact composition of which is usually unknown. Fungi are usually grown at 25°C, at which temperature they generally take around seven days to grow. In contrast, viruses are far more difficult to grow in the laboratory and must either be grown in the host or in what is called tissue culture, a technique which involves the use of living fragments of animal or plant tissue or separated cells which have been removed from the whole organism.

The science of microbiology largely developed from the study of bacteria which cause infections in humans and animals. As more and more microorganisms were discovered, and their role in nature determined, the subject began to widen and fragment. Today micro-biologists can specialize in the study of medical microbiology, microbial physiology or genetics and microbial ecology. They can also specialize in the study of one group of microorganisms with the result that the science of microbiology is now divided into the study of bacteriology, mycology (the study of fungi), virology, algology, and protozoology. Unfortunately, the obvious end result of this specialization is that bacteriologists, for example, often know little about how to identify fungi, while mycologists often restrict themselves purely to the study of moulds. An unfortunate outcome in the recent developments in molecular biology, the biggest breakthroughs in which have stemmed from studies in bacterial genetics, is that large numbers of microbiology students are now specializing in this one area, and most of the new academic posts in universities throughout the world are being filled with microbial geneticists or molecular biologists. While there is no doubting the fundamental importance of these subjects, it is likely that in the not too distant future there will arise a marked shortage of microbiologists who are specialists in, for example, microbial taxonomy, ecology and physiology. Such a dearth of non-molecular microbiologists is likely to have a major deleterious impact on future studies of aetiology (i.e. factors influencing the spread of pathogens), ecology, and physiology of pathogenic microorganisms.

ANTIBIOTICS DEFINED

What exactly are antibiotics? My family dictionary gives the following definition: 'Drugs from living organisms which prevent the growth and reproduction of other organisms'. This definition, although similar to the original given by Selman Waksman, the co-discoverer of strepto-mycin, differs in several important details. Waksman's definition was 'A compound produced by one microorganism which is capable of killing or inhibiting another'. Thus the original definition of the word antibiotic is restricted to a compound produced by and which affects only microorganisms. Strictly speaking then, an antibiotic cannot be produced by, say, an animal or higher plant. Despite this, however, antimicrobial compounds have been described as antibiotics, even when they are from such diverse sources as lichens, plants and insects. Waksman did not approve of this loose use of his terminology. He originally coined the word antibiotic in early 1942, when Dr J. E. Flynn, the Editor of *Biological Abstracts* (a journal providing a source of abstracts of biological literature), asked him to suggest a word to describe the various antimicrobial compounds which were then beginning to appear with increasing frequency in the medical-scientific literature. Waksman provided the word antibiotic, a variant of 'anti-biosis', which had long been in use to describe the antagonistic effect which some microorganisms exhibit towards others. Burkholder, another antibiotic pioneer, argued, however, that the term 'antibiotic' had in fact been coined in 1889, and was used as recently as 1928. Despite this, Waksman is generally regarded as the man who originated the modern definition, which reached *Index Medicus* in 1943, and soon became generally accepted. It was not without its critics, however. Howard Florey, for one, objected to the word because, taken literally, it meant 'against life' and clearly, he argued, a substance that could snatch a person from the 'jaws of death' is not best described in this way. Florey appears to have preferred the word 'bacteriostat', while other alter-natives which never caught on included 'antibiotin' and 'antisymbiotic'.

Waksman stoutly defended his original definition of the word antibiotic against the many attempts to corrupt it. An excellent example was recently given by Dr David Pramer, who had been one of Waksman's research students. He relates how Waksman took a speaker to task at a scientific meeting for his reference to antitumour antibiotics. Pramer, who is now head of the Institute which bears Waksman's name, rose somewhat sheepishly and asked his former mentor, 'If the use of the word antibiotic is to be limited to substances of microbial origin that are active against other microbes, then what would you suggest be used to describe a substance of microbial origin that is active against cancer?'. Waksman, who was well versed in the art of scientific in-fighting, waited a moment, sighed and then wearily waved his hand. 'Pramer,' he said, 'first you find something that is active against cancer and then I will tell you what to call it!'

'MAGIC BULLETS': A PRELUDE TO ANTIBIOTICS

Strictly speaking then, the term antibiotic refers only to the products of microbial metabolism which are used to treat microbial disease, particularly when caused by bacteria. There are, however, a number of chemically synthesized compounds which, although they can be used to the same effect, are not what Waksman would have termed antibiotics.

The first of these compounds appeared long before the antibiotics, but had a similarly profound effect on medicine. They are often referred to as 'magic bullets' because of their seemingly magical effect on certain bacterial infections, and because, like a bullet, they are targeted, in this case, towards a specific pathogen.

Salvarsan was the first of the 'magic bullets'. Appearing in the summer of 1910, it caused considerable excitement because of its ability to cure syphilis. So great was the demand for this new drug that the factory in the town of Hoechst near Frankfurt was besieged by patients and doctors alike, all hoping to obtain a sample of this life-saving, dye-like compound. Unfortunately, the limited supplies of salvarsan had to be reserved for clinical trials, and such was the risk of them being stolen that the results of the daily production run were carefully monitored and then deposited in one of the company's safes.

Salvarsan was discovered by the German chemist, Paul Erlich, aided by an assistant called Sachachiro Hata. Erlich was one of the brilliant young men who was attracted to work in Robert Koch's laboratory during the 1880s. Here he soon made a name for himself by developing a stain which allowed bacteriologists for the first time to see clearly the tubercle bacillus under the microscope, an approach which was later modified as a test for the presence of the pathogen in sputum.

In 1901, Erlich became interested in the work of one Alphonse Laveran, who had been trying to kill trypanosome parasites (the cause of sleeping sickness) which he had injected into mice. At that time Erlich was not interested in curing syphilis, but when Fritz Schaudinn showed that this disease was caused by a trypanosome-like organism (*Treponema pallida*), he immediately began to search for an arsenic compound which might cure the age-old scourge of the 'pox'.

Shortly before the turn of the century, Erlich moved from Berlin to head the Institute for Experimental Therapy in Frankfurt. Near here was located the Hoechst Dye Works, where the head of pharmacy was August Laubenheimer, a former Professor of Chemistry in Giessen.

Erlich had come to the conclusion that it should be possible to synthesize chemical compounds capable of inhibiting bacteria, but without damaging body cells. So impressed were the Hoechst company scientists by these ideas that they decided to devote a large part of the resources of their pharmacy department to help find such novel antibacterial agents.

Erlich began by evaluating the antibacterial properties of methylene blue, a dye first synthesized by Hoechst in 1885. Over a period of five years, he worked with this compound, aided by a Japanese assistant, K. Shiga, but no cure was found, and the thousands of rats and mice sacrificed in the experiments appeared to have died in vain.

From 1906 onwards, Erlich concentrated his reseach on finding a cure for syphilis. His efforts were initially directed towards the arsenic compound, atoxyl, but when this compound was found to severely damage the central nervous system the hunt began for new and less toxic arsenic derivatives. Limited success was achieved with compounds like arsenophyl glycine and acetyl arsenilate, but it was clear that a more thorough search would have to be made of the countless arsenic compounds then being synthesized by Hoechst. To help him with this laborious testing programme, Erlich employed Hata, another Japanese scientist. Soon, thousands of experimental animals were again being sacrificed in the search for a cure for syphilis. This time they were not to die in vain.

By the time arsenic compound number 592 had been reached the normally imperturbable Hata was extremely excited. This compound, diaminodioxyarsenobenzol, while toxic, proved highly inhibitory towards the syphilis spirochaete. The compound was then purified and made more soluble, and the result, preparation 606, or Salvarsan, was to become the most famous numbered compound in medicine.

The first humans to receive 606 (also called arsphenamine) were treated by Professor Konrad Alt. Although the results were near miraculous they were soon improved upon by the appearance of a variant of Salvarsan called Neosalvarsan, a compound which was water soluble, and, since it contained only 19 per cent arsenic, was far less toxic than earlier arsenic compounds. Within five years of the first widespread use of this compound the incidence of syphilis in England and France was halved!

Salvarsan was far from ideal as a chemotherapeutic agent. For one thing, it was so dangerous that a dose could only be given every seven days. It also came as a dry, largely insoluble powder, and it had to be dissolved in 600 cc of water literally at the patient's bedside. It was then given intravenously. If any escaped from the vein, it could cause necrosis leading to the loss of the arm! Rashes might develop and the liver become so damaged that the patient would become jaundiced. Such treatment would continue for at least a year before a cure could be pronounced.

Unfortunately, the extensive use of Salvarsan often led to its misuse, which brought about a feeling of revulsion amongst some physicians. It was a toxic drug when given in large doses, and much of Erlich's time was spent in demonstrating how it could be safely given without causing adverse effects or even death. Some even questioned whether Salvarsan was of sufficient value in syphilis treatment to compensate for its untoward effects. Others even doubted that it was any better than mercury, and, as late as 1914, the prestigious *Journal of the American Medical Association* questioned its value as an adequate substitute for mercury in the treatment of syphilis. Some, like Professor Gaucher of Paris University, went further, describing it as the 'German Poison'! Nevertheless, doctors continued to persevere with Salvarsan, until eventually they found that in correct doses, spread over long periods, the new drug could indeed safely defeat syphilis.

Once syphilis had been conquered it was assumed that bacterial infection as a whole would fall prey to the 'magic bullets'. But unfortunately Salvarsan was to prove effective only against this single, albeit important, disease. Despite this, new chemical compounds continued to be tested for their antibacterial properties in the vain hope that a more versatile 'magic bullet' might be found.

The most active group involved in this search during the 1930s was employed by another German chemical firm, the giant dye company, I. G. Farben Industrie. Here, a large staff of chemists was employed to synthesize dyes. These were then passed on to Gerhard Domagk, whose group tested them for any antibacterial properties. Domagk was head of the Company's Institute for Experimental Pathology at Elberfield. In the autumn of 1932, he received a bright red dye for testing which proved to be remarkably effective in curing mice which had been infected with pathogenic streptococci. This new compound, named Prontosil, would at last provide medical science with a means of combating a wide range of bacterial infections.

It would be another three years before Prontosil, after being fully protected by patents, was released for general use. Strangely, this new compound proved effective only when injected into a test animal or patient, and would not kill bacteria in culture. It was later shown that the effectiveness of Prontosil resulted from the activity of a component of the molecule, the sulphonamide moiety, which was released in the body as a degradation product. As a result it was the sulphonamides, rather than Prontosil, which would eventually have such a major impact on the treatment of infectious disease.

One of the first patients to receive Prontosil was Domagk's own daughter, who had contracted a dangerous streptococcal infection after pricking her finger with a needle. Fortunately, a large dose of the new antibacterial saved her life. Much later, the life of Winston Churchill was saved by the injection of a sulphonamide. This famous incident took place in Carthage, just after the Teheran Conference. Churchill began to suffer from a sore throat and chest pains which then developed into pneumonia. His personal physician, Lord Moran, asked the help of an army surgeon called Pulvertaft who, as we shall see, did some pioneering work with both the crude form of penicillin and later the purified product. Pulvertaft was in favour of using penicillin to treat Churchill, but Moran insisted that a sulphonamide be used instead of penicillin which was then something of an experimental drug. Nevertheless, in popular mythology, it was penicillin, rather than the sulpha drugs, which saved Churchill's life. It is ironic that these compounds which were the product of the German pharmaceutical industry should have had such a dramatic effect in determining the course of the Second World War.

The sulphonamides were to prove particularly useful in the treatment of puerperal fever. Before the appearance of these compounds this disease, which is also known as childbed or lying-in fever was one of the most intractable diseases known. It was particularly distressing because it often resulted in the death of the mother soon after giving birth.

As early as 1795, the Aberdeen doctor, Alexander Gordon, had suggested that puerperal fever only infected mothers who had been examined by doctors or midwives, a conclusion to be also arrived at in 1843 by Oliver Wendell Holmes. Conclusive proof that doctors were frequently involved in transmitting this infection resulted from some famous experiments conducted in Vienna by Ignaz Semmelweis. In 1846, Semmelweis became an assistant in obstetrics at the Allgemeines Krankenhaus in Vienna. There were two maternity wards in the hospital, one used to train medical students while the other was devoted to the education of nurses and midwives. Semmelweis noticed that the death rate amongst mothers was highest in the ward attended by students, and, even more importantly, fell off during their vacations. He realized that the students were inspecting their patients straight after working in the autopsy room, and as a result were presumably passing on the infection from the cadavers to the mothers! By forcing the students to wash their hands in a chlorine solution Semmelweis dramatically reduced the incidence of puerperal fever in the student ward. The first students to wash their hands in chlorine water did so in May 1874. As the solution had an acrid smell, was unpleasant to work with, and was also expensive, it was soon replaced by chlorinated lime which fortunately turned out to have the same disinfectant effect. The results were staggering. In the last seven months of 1847, Semmelweis's methods reduced the mortality from 11 per cent down to 3 per cent, and by 1848, for the first time in history, mortality in the teaching clinic fell below that in the midwives' ward. There were setbacks however. In one case a woman was admitted into the labour ward suffering from a bad ulcer on her left knee joint. There was no reason why the infection should spread to her womb. Yet, despite all precautions with hand washing, the infection spread and caused a number of deaths. Semmelweis concluded, in somewhat florid language, that: 'The air of the labour room loaded with the putrid matter, found its way into the gaping genitals just at the completion of labour, and onward into the cavity of the uterus where the putrid matter was absorbed, and puerperal fever was the consequence.' Despite this setback, mortality rates in the ward employing his methods eventually fell to as low as 1.3 per cent.

In 1857, Semmelweis published his findings in a book called *Aetiology, Conception and Prophylaxis of Childbed Fever*, which took him all of three years to write. It was a long, rambling and repetitive, egotistical work which emphasized his belief that he had been subjected to continued persecution for his ideas. Not surprisingly, the book met with ridicule. Semmelweis's behaviour became increasingly eccentric and by 1865 it was clear that he was suffering from a mental illness. He died insane in 1865, a victim of a bacterial infection of the hand, an unsung pioneer who had dared to question the methods employed by the medical profession. On his death, Semmelweis's body was taken back to the Vienna General Hospital. Here an autopsy showed that he had been suffering from extensive brain damage.

By the early 1930s, the source of puerperal fever was well established, but still the disease was incurable. Then, in 1936, Leonard Colebrook demonstrated the value of Prontosil. Interestingly, the first person to be treated by Colebrook was not a puerperal fever sufferer, but one of his colleagues, Ronald Hare. We will hear more of Hare later, because of his involvement in the penicillin story. In January 1936, Hare pricked his finger with a sliver of glass infected with streptococci. He became critically ill and was in danger of losing his arm if not his life. Colebrook administered Prontosil almost as a last resort. The first result was that Hare turned bright pink, an unpleasant side effect of the fact that Prontosil was a dye! Fortunately, the treatment proved a complete success, and helped convince Colebrook that Prontosil was worthy of further investigation. Ronald Hare's response when he first heard of Prontosil is interesting because it shows how little faith doctors had at that time in the concept of intravenous therapy; 'My first reaction was to throw the postcard [written by a contact in Paris] down with the thought "another of those damned compounds with a trade name and of unknown composition that are of no use anyway" . . . We were time and time again infuriated by the claims put forward by clinicians and commercial firms for compounds that should never have been introduced at all.'

A second early use of Prontosil by Colebrook involved the treatment of one of his technicians, W. R. Maxted. Maxted acquired a very severe tonsillitis from conducting experimental work with streptococci and Colebrook decided to use Prontosil to try and cure it. The particular strain of *Streptococcus* involved was apparently very virulent and there was every likelihood that the infection would become life-threatening. On receiving Prontosil, Maxted reported an awful feeling in his stomach, and an intense internal heat, which made him feel as if he were about to die! Despite being violently sick, Maxted was cured, and he was able to return to his experimental work on the streptococci. In the sixty-four cases of puerperal fever which Colebrook then treated with Prontosil the death rate was cut from the usual 25 per cent to a mere 5 per cent. No one could now doubt that the long awaited 'chemotherapeutic age' had at last dawned.

In 1938, sulphonamide compounds like M and B 693 (sulphapyridine), produced by May and Baker, appeared, whose first success was to cure a Norfolk labourer who was suffering from severe pneumonia. By 1941 compounds like these were in widespread use, and some two thousand tons of sulphonamides had been administered to some ten to fifteen million people! Yet the impact of these compounds on medicine is now largely forgotten. The sulphonamides saved countless lives, however. They were used to good effect by the Americans after the Japanese bombing of Pearl Harbour, while the Axis powers had to rely upon them throughout the course of the last War.

Gerhard Domagk, the discoverer of Prontosil, was awarded the Nobel Prize in 1939 but, because of one of Hitler's fits of pique, was unable to accept it. He retired from research work as late as 1960, but after being dogged by rheumatic fever, he died in 1964. His gift to medicine saved many lives and also had a profound effect on medical scientific thought. Before Prontosil, the idea that by injecting a compound one might cure generalized bacterial infection was largely ridiculed. Prontosil showed it could be done, and the way was open for the rediscovery of penicillin, and the beginning of the golden age of antibiotics.

2

The Discovery of Penicillin

The discovery of penicillin ranks as one of the most important in the history of medicine. It was the first, and remains the most important, of the antibiotics. It revolutionized medicine and largely removed the scourge of once killer diseases such as pneumonia, puerperal fever, bacterial meningitis and staphylococcal septicaemia.

Penicillin was discovered by Alexander Fleming in 1928. Fleming was later to receive worldwide acclaim for the discovery and is still generally regarded as the man who gave penicillin to the world. However, while Fleming undoubtedly discovered penicillin, and was the first to try and use it to cure infections, his attempts to achieve the all important purification were largely unsuccessful. Nor did he achieve the first cures with penicillin, an accolade which fell to one of his former students, Cecil G. Paine, who did his work independently of Fleming at the Royal Infirmary in Sheffield during 1929–30.

The miraculous therapeutic powers of penicillin were to remain unrecognized, however, until around 1940, when it was purified by a team of Oxford University scientists led by Howard Florey. The development of penicillin then moved to the USA, where scientists were to be remarkably successful at producing large quantities of cheap penicillin just in time to treat Allied soldiers, from D-day onwards.

The discovery and subsequent development of penicillin is one of the most remarkable stories to emerge from the history of medical and scientific research. Its appearance encouraged scientists to search for new antimicrobial agents which then entered the physician's armoury.

Most readers will be familiar with at least the outline of how penicillin was discovered. In the popular version of the story, a mould spore is said to have blown in through Fleming's laboratory window and alighted on some bacteriological growth medium contained in a

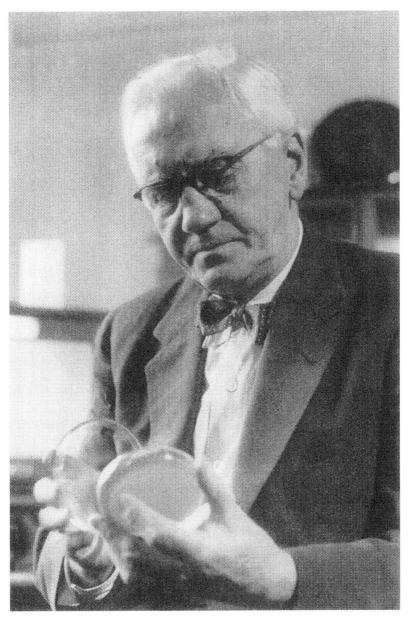

Plate 1   Alexander Fleming, the discoverer of penicillin.
(© St Mary's Hospital)

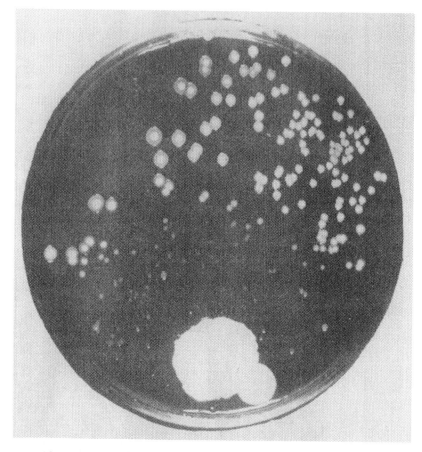

Plate 2 Fleming's famous plate, showing the contaminating mould
lysing colonies of *Staph. aureus* as well as forming a distinct zone of
inhibition. (© St Mary's Hospital)

glass petri dish. This mould then grew and inhibited some colonies of
pathogenic bacteria which Fleming had seeded onto the medium. It was
then grown in large quantities and purified into the life-saving drug that
we know today. Unfortunately this simplified account of penicillin's
discovery is full of half truths and inaccuracies which tend to have the
effect of trivializing one of the most fascinating discoveries in medical
history.

   How then did Fleming come to discover this, the first and most
famous of the antibiotics, and what trials did it have to endure before it
became established in medicine?

On the morning of either the third or fourth of September 1928, Fleming returned to his laboratory at St Mary's Hospital, London, from Suffolk, where he had been on holiday at his country retreat. This was to be a flying visit, in response to a plea for assistance from a colleague, who was treating a patient with a bad abscess. As he sat at his bench, Fleming began to sort through some petri dishes containing a bacterio-logical growth medium (referred to by bacteriologists as plates). There are two different accounts of what happened next. In the first, related by David Masters in his superb, if short, account of the penicillin story, called *Miracle Drug*, Fleming picked up the plate which he had left incubating on the bench. Then he noticed something and turned to Dr E. W. Todd, with whom he shared the laboratory, and said, 'Now look at this, this is very interesting. I like this sort of thing – it might be very important.'

A slightly different account of what happened that morning is given by Ronald Hare in *The Birth of Penicillin*, and by Gwyn MacFarlane in his recent biography of Fleming. According to this interpretation of the events, Fleming was found sorting through plates not by Todd, but by D. M. Pryce, a research scholar at St Mary's. These plates were not picked up from the bench, as described in the first account, but had been left high and dry in a tray of a disinfectant called lysol. This time Fleming is reported to have uttered the words 'That's funny!'

Now these two accounts of the penicillin discovery, while essentially similar, differ in a number of important respects. Apart from the obvious disagreement as to the identity of the other person present, the significant difference between the accounts is that in the version given by Masters, Fleming seems to have purposely left the plates on the bench; while in the Hare-MacFarlane account they had been dumped in dis-infectant. Masters appears to have inherited his version from Dr Todd, while the alternative account was originally related by Price and was cor-roborated by another St Mary's man, Dr S. T. Craddock, of whom we will hear more later. Fleming's own account of the discovery would, however, appear to support the Masters account of what happened.

Fleming's photograph of the famous plate which he picked up that morning shows a distinct fungal colony surrounded by numerous bacterial colonies. In the vicinity of the mould colony these bacteria (*Staphylococcus aureus*) are dramatically reduced in number and acquire a transparent look, forming what Fleming referred to as 'ghosts'. Clearly the mould was causing the bacteria to lyse or dissolve. Now colonies of *Staphylococcus* are notoriously difficult to lyse, so when he saw the penicillin effect Fleming's curiosity was immediately aroused. Some years earlier, he had discovered lysozyme, a similar lytic agent which is present in body fluids. Lysozyme dissolves only some bacteria which do not cause infections, and so found no use in medicine. In the case of penicillin, however, Fleming was confronted with the lysis of a medically important pathogen, which causes infections ranging from simple boils to the fatal poisoning of the blood stream, or septicaemia. It is clear that it was lysis, rather than mere bacterial inhibition, which attracted Fleming's attention when he discovered penicillin. This is why his role in the discovery was so pivotal; anyone else might have overlooked this lysis, but Fleming had seen something of the like before. His was 'the prepared mind' which Pasteur had said nature so much favours.

We have a detailed account of Fleming's first impressions of penicillin. This was given on 20 February 1946 in a lecture to the staff of the Mayo Clinic and later published in their Staff Meeting Proceedings under the title, 'Antiseptics Old and New'. He describes his work as follows:

> I need not go into details of the research on which I was engaged at the time but my culture plate was covered with staphylococcal colonies. The particular work involved opening the plate and looking at it under a dissecting microscope and then leaving it for growth to take place. That, of course, was asking for trouble by contamination, as things were always dropping from the air and sure enough, trouble came but it led to penicillin. A mould spore, coming from I don't know where, dropped on the plate. That didn't excite me. I had seen such contamination before, but what I had never seen before was staphylococci undergoing lysis around the contaminating colony. Obviously something extraordinary was happening.

The fact that it was bacterial lysis, rather than merely inhibition, which caught Fleming's eye is further emphasized by the following statement which he made at a meeting of the Royal Society of Medicine in November 1943: 'It was no new thing for a bacteriologist to find that a mould had grown on a culture plate which had lain on the bench for a week, but the strange thing in this particular case was that the bacterial colonies in the neighbourhood of the mould appeared to be fading away.'

Although Fleming tried to repeat these initial observations, he was unable to get the mould to induce the lysis which had so interested him. Nevertheless, he soon found that penicillin's ability to prevent the growth of certain bacteria was in itself exciting.

Microbiologists in Fleming's day were well aware that many of the organisms which they studied could inhibit the growth of their neighbours. Such antagonism was, however, generally explained by assuming that one organism denied the other nutrients or perhaps changed the pH of the medium, making it an unfavourable environment for the growth of the other. Fleming, on the other hand, realized that his contaminating mould must be excreting an antibacterial agent, which if it could be extracted and purified might play an important role in the fight against infection.

Ronald Hare, a bacteriologist who worked in the same department at St Mary's as Fleming, has recently tried to replicate the steps necessary for penicillin to be discovered in the way that Fleming did. While it was easy for Hare to demonstrate bacterial inhibition, attempts to replicate lysis ended in failure. The explanation for this apparent anomaly is quite complex. In the early 1940s it was found that penicillin was incapable of inhibiting fully formed bacterial cells, but instead only inhibited them while in the process of producing new cell walls and dividing. Now growth inhibition and lysis are not the same thing, and penicillin's bacteriolytic effect occurs under a variety of complex conditions. Hare has suggested that Fleming inoculated his plates with bacteria, at which point they became contaminated with airborne fungal spores. The mould then grew and produced penicillin, while the growth of the bacterium was held back by the relatively low room temperature. The room temperature then increased, allowing the bacteria to divide and grow, but those colonies close to the mould culture were inhibited by the penicillin. Hare, by checking meteorological records, demonstrated that the temperature conditions prevailing in London during September 1928 were exactly right to allow this series of events to occur. Unfortunately, Hare's experiments do not explain the appearance of bacterial lysis, nor in fact do they accurately replicate what Fleming was doing when he discovered penicillin.

Is there, then, an alternative explanation to account for how Fleming came to observe the penicillin effect? To answer this question we have to take a detailed look at the work which Fleming was doing which led to the discovery.

Fleming was a recognized authority on medically important bacteria, and in 1928 he was asked to write a review on the staphylococci. The resulting paper appeared in the second volume of *A System of Bacteriology in Relation to Medicine*, which was published by the Medical Research Council. That Fleming concentrated on his mould's ability to lyse bacteria is further emphasized by the following comment which he makes on page 15 of this review: 'A common laboratory contaminant, a *Penicillium*, has a very marked lytic action on staphylococci growing in its neighbourhood.'

In order to do the review justice, it was necessary for Fleming to read all the available literature on these bacteria. It was while searching this literature that Fleming came across a report originating from the School of Pathology at Trinity College in Dublin. Written by Joseph Bigger and his colleagues, this paper described how colonies of *Staphylococcus* took on unusual morphologies when incubated under non-standard temperature conditions. The standard condition for growing these bacteria is to leave them overnight at 37°C. Bigger's work involved leaving these bacteria to grow for long periods at a variety of incubation conditions, including room temperature.

Fleming, clearly intrigued by Bigger's paper, was attempting to repeat the work just prior to going off on his summer holidays. The opening line of his first penicillin paper states as much: 'While working with staphylococcal variants a number of culture plates were set aside on the laboratory bench and examined from time to time.' Set aside does not, as is often assumed, mean that the plates were left haphazardly, but that they were put on the side to incubate at room temperature. In some cases, Fleming probably incubated the plates for short periods at higher temperatures, in order to induce culture variants. This short incubation at relatively high temperature may have stimulated the staphylococcal colonies to develop, but not to the point where they became visible to the naked eye. Fleming would then have checked the surface of the medium using a hand lens and it could have been at this point, rather than at the time of inoculation, that the mould contamination occurred. The mould could then have developed at room temperature and produced penicillin. As Hare has pointed out, the room temperature might then have increased, at which point growth and then lysis may have occurred. Two months before he died, in 1955, Fleming gave an interview to the BBC in which he made the following comment about the penicillin discovery: 'I got contamination, all sorts of contamination; one of them, a mould, produced penicillin.' Fleming's reference here to 'all sorts' of microbial contamination is interesting because it is unlikely that a bacteriologist as experienced as he was would have suffered such extensive contamination, unless, that is, he was involved in doing something unusual. The unusual work in this case was to remove the petri dish lid and to observe young colonies of staphylococci using a hand lens, a process which would inevitably lead to the surface of the nutrient medium being exposed to the air and, as a result, a wide variety of contaminants, one of which turned out to be the penicillin-producing mould.

In the popular account of Fleming's discovery, the mould is said to have entered his laboratory from Praed Street below. A glance back at the Mayo Clinic quote of Fleming's which is given above will convince the reader that Fleming, at least initially, was unaware of the origin of the contaminating mould spores. Now the atmosphere around us is teeming with fungal spores and it is quite possible that a spore of a *Penicillium* could have blown into Fleming's laboratory from the street below. However, it is equally likely that the spore could have originated from the air inside the building. It turns out that it is very unlikely that Fleming's laboratory window could have been the port of entry of the spores. This is quite simply because no self-respecting or, for that matter, self-preserving bacteriologist would work with open windows, for fear that he or she might become infected with the pathogenic bacteria being handled. Fleming had devoted his life's work to the study of bacteria and good sterile technique was second nature to him, so he would never have had the window open while inoculating his plates. There is an even more prosaic reason why the window was unlikely to have been open when the plates were contaminated, namely that it was difficult to open, although this could apparently be achieved with the aid of a system of ropes and pulleys.

If the window was not the entry port of the mould spores, then where did they originate from? Again Ronald Hare's detective work has provided us with a likely explanation. It seems that the spores originated not from Praed Street, but from the laboratory below Fleming's room which was occupied by a young mycologist called C. J. La Touche. This young man had recently been busy collecting isolates of fungi from all over London, in an attempt to show that they were involved in causing asthma. Despite La Touche's best efforts, it is likely that the spores of some of his fungi contaminated the air of his own laboratory and were then carried upstairs to where Fleming was working. Hare has even provided convincing evidence to suggest that the spores were carried between the laboratories by the connecting shaft of a dumbwaiter which linked the rooms.

Since Fleming's penicillin-producing mould is not a particularly common member of the spore population of non-laboratory air it appears more than likely that his contaminating culture originated from La Touche's culture collection. One piece of evidence tends to confirm this likelihood. After Fleming had discovered penicillin, he was naturally interested to find out if it was produced by fungi other than his contaminate. As he was not an expert on moulds he had no cultures of fungi of his own and so borrowed a few from La Touche. Fleming found that none of these cultures produced penicillin, with one exception, a culture which had exactly the same cultural and morphological characteristics as Fleming's isolate. So it is likely that La Touche's isolate and the penicillin-producer were one and the same.

There is one final version of how Fleming came to discover penicillin, one which involves far less of an element of chance than does the generally accepted story. This theory was first suggested by a bacteriologist called D. B. Colquhoun. It was his contention that Fleming did not discover penicillin by accident but, instead, purposely inoculated bacteria onto a plate already contaminated with a fungus. Whether the mould had arrived by accident or was grown specifically for the purpose is not made clear by Colquhoun. The theory has a number of convenient advantages over the standard account of the discovery. In particular, it helps avoid the complications referred to above regarding the fact that the penicillin effect can only be produced if the mould grows before the bacterium which it inhibits. The main drawback with this theory would appear to be that no self-respecting bacteriologist would inoculate bacteria onto an already contaminated plate. Colquhoun, however, states that he himself had often inoculated bacteria onto culture plates, particularly of blood agar, which he knew to be contaminated with a small mould colony. He then goes on to suggest that Fleming knew from his reading of the literature what to expect, or that perhaps he inoculated the contaminated plate merely to see what would happen. Colquhoun makes reference to the following quote by Fleming to support his theory: 'My occupation is a simple one – I play with microbes. There are of course many rules in the play, and a certain amount of knowledge is required before you can fully enjoy the game but when you have acquired knowledge and experience, it is very pleasant to break the rules and to be able to find something which no one has ever thought of.'

Fleming was probably being characteristically dismissive of his work when he made these comments: they certainly fall far short of evidence in support of Colquhoun's hypothesis. Firstly, there is nothing in the early literature to suggest that a certain species of penicillin might produce a compound as effective at killing bacteria as is penicillin. As we shall see, there were numerous reports of antagonism between *Penicillium* species and bacteria in the early literature, but Fleming would have been faced with the prospect of screening thousands of isolates before he came across a penicillin producer. Secondly, it is likely that he would have been quite happy to have admitted the higher degree of scientific forethought implied in Colquhoun's account of the discovery.

Ernst Chain's views on how penicillin came to be discovered are worth considering since they emphasize the importance of lysis, but also make a tantalizing reference to the possibility that Colquhoun's ideas are more plausible than they first appear. In 1971, Chain read a paper at a meeting sponsored by the Royal Society and the Royal College of

Physicians to celebrate the thirtieth anniversary of the first clinical use of penicillin, in which he made the following statement:

> The unusual element in Fleming's case was that he left his petri dish with the staphylococci colonies on its agar for such a long time on the bench that the contaminating mould had time to develop and to exert its antibacterial action on the colonies, and that the colonies were just at the right age and physiological state in which they underwent autolysis under the influence of penicillin. Fleming did not discover the growth-inhibiting effect of penicillin on bacteria directly by observing a phenomenon of inhibition of bacterial growth (which penicillin commonly exerts on many bacterial species under many growth conditions and which is, of course, the basis of its chemotherapeutic action) but through a bacterio-lytic effect of penicillin which it exerts only under very special conditions not normally encountered in the bacterio-logical laboratory and only on a very few bacterial species. Fortunately the *Staphylococcus* on which Fleming had worked was amongst these. The reason that the antibacterial action of penicillin on bacteria was not discovered long before Fleming despite its ubiquitous occurrence, was that normally if the bacteriologist sees that one of his plates which he wishes to use for a diagnostic test is contaminated with a mould he does not use it, and thus has no chance of observing an inhibition of bacterial growth by the con-taminant: on the other hand once his bacteriological observation is completed, he throws away the Petri dishes as soon as possible without waiting for contamination to appear.

Chain seems to me to be implying here that Fleming did actually streak bacteria onto a plate which was already contaminated by the penicillin-producing mould, in the way suggested by Colquhoun. What evidence he has for this view is, however, not made clear.

With the help of a student, Martin Haddock, I recently attempted like the late Ronald Hare, to repeat Fleming's 'accidental' discovery of penicillin. I was particularly eager that we should demonstrate, in as random a fashion as possible, the lytic action of *P. notatum* on *Staphylococcus aureus*. To do this, we transferred Fleming's original fungus to Czapek Dox or meat extract media in petri dishes. When the mould began to produce large numbers of spores the dish was placed, with the lid removed, in a plastic container. Within a few hours the air inside was filled with spores. We hoped that a fungal spore would fall on the medium and produce a contaminant which would be analogous to that seen by Fleming. The method worked surprisingly well, and we were next able to test for the presence of penicillin by spreading a culture of *Staphylococcus aureus* onto the artificially contaminated medium. We then incubated these plates at various temperatures for varying periods of time, in order to replicate the kind of conditions that Fleming might have used had he been attempting to reproduce Bigger's work on bacterial variants. Like Hare before us, we found it very easy to show that *P. notatum* has an inhibitory effect on *Staphylococcus aureus*, but despite using some eighty variations in temperature and exposure lengths we simply could not produce the bacterial lysis which had so attracted Fleming's attention. So while the inhibitory effect of *P. notatum* may frequently have been observed prior to Fleming's observations, the all important lytic action was an extremely rare occurrence. Can we explain why this lytic effect is so difficult to reproduce? One possibility is that Fleming's isolate has mutated over the years, and has lost the ability to produce a lytic agent, which may in fact have been something other than penicillin. It is also possible that the strain of *Staphylococcus* which he was using was far more prone to lysis than the one that both we and Hare used. Perhaps the answer to this intriguing question will never be found, and we will have to be content with marvelling at the sheer improbability of the events which conspired to present Fleming with the phenomenon, an opportunity of which he took full advantage. For the moment we must be satisfied to accept that penicillin was discovered in the way that Fleming described. It was fortuitous, but it relied on the involvement of an investigator with a keen eye as well as a prepared mind.

Fleming's observations would have led nowhere had he not acted upon them. It would have been easy for him to have observed the penicillin effect and then set the plate to one side while he attended to what seemed more pressing work. His first step was to produce large quantities of his 'mould juice', to enable him to study its properties in more detail, and perhaps to purify the active ingredient. If Fleming had expected this last task to be straightforward then he was disappointed. In fact, the purification step would always elude him.

Fleming spent much of the autumn of 1928 busily finding out what he could about the new substance. In the process, he took two crucial steps. Firstly he had the mould identified and secondly he wrote a paper in which the results of his studies were given in some detail. To help him in identifying the mould he enlisted the help of La Touche, whose property, I have suggested, it originally was. La Touche was doubtless very busy in the time-consuming job of identifying his own fungal isolates. He was, therefore, probably not overjoyed when a senior scientist from upstairs added yet another culture to his collection of unknowns. Not surprisingly, La Touche seems to have given the culture only a cursory look before he pronounced it to be a strain of *Penicillium rubrum*. Fleming, apparently, was not particularly happy with this identification, but accepted it on the basis of the younger man's superior knowledge of fungi.

Fleming's doubts proved sound. In fact, mycologists and medical historians have long wondered what induced La Touche to make this apparently obvious error in identification. This is because *P. rubrum*, unlike Fleming's mould, produces a vivid red pigment from which it derives its specific name. Why did an experienced mycologist like La Touche pronounce Fleming's isolate to be a 'red penicillium'? The answer is quite simple: Fleming's isolate did originally produce a red pigment, a characteristic which it has since lost, presumably as the result of repeated transfer onto fresh growth media. We know this is the case, because Fleming informs us of the fact on the first page of his famous paper. La Touche wrote a letter to Fleming on 3 November 1945, some time after penicillin had become famous, apologizing for his error as follows:

> As I know that you accepted this nomenclature against your better judgement perhaps you will allow me to write to Dr Herrell stating what I know to be the truth. I think you will remember that it was your opinion at the time that the mould was *P. chrysogenum*. I regret very much that at the time I did not make a more thorough investigation and am very sorry indeed to have thus misled you into publishing an incorrect statement in your original paper. I trust that this letter makes clear, although perhaps belatedly, that the responsibility for this mistake is entirely my own.

La Touche's misidentification was not as damaging as it might have been, because Fleming had the foresight to deposit the culture with the collection held by the Medical Research Council. So even if it had been wrongly named it was still available to anyone who wanted a sample. In the event, the isolate was given its correct name, *Penicillium notatum*, before it was accepted into the collection. On the other hand, the error might have caused problems if anyone had hoped to replicate Fleming's findings using *P. rubrum* (which does not produce penicillin) rather than a subculture of Fleming's isolate.

The second important decision which Fleming made was to publish a paper on his penicillin work. This he submitted to the *British Journal Of*

Experimental Pathology on 10 May 1929, and it was published in the tenth volume of the Journal which appeared in June of the same year.

In this paper, Fleming summarizes the results of his studies on penicillin. He reported the cultural conditions which promoted the growth of the mould and encouraged it to produce penicillin. Next, he informed the reader that penicillin had a selective effect on bacteria. Fleming had put this selective inhibition to good effect by using penicillin-amended media to isolate certain pathogens from infected patients. While penicillin inhibited a number of pathogenic bacteria it had no effect on Pfeiffer's bacillus, which was then widely but incorrectly thought to cause influenza. As a result of this selective inhibition, the bacillus could be isolated even from a mixed bacteria obtained, for example, from a throat swab. Fleming also pointed out that penicillin had a marked inhibitory effect on pyogenic cocci (such as those causing boils), and the diphtheria bacillus, but it did not inhibit either the coli-typhoid group, enterococci. Fleming then devoted his attention to the attempts which had been made in his laboratory to isolate pure penicillin, and commented on its solubility in a variety of solvents. He went on to make the point that the crude material is non-irritant to body tissue, and does not inhibit the vital functioning of the white blood corpuscles. Finally, and perhaps most importantly, Fleming made reference to the possible clinical use of penicillin in the following words: 'It is suggested that it may be an efficient antiseptic for application to, or injection into, areas affected by penicillin sensitive microbes.' Here, Fleming was clearly referring to the potential medical use of penicillin, although it is not certain that he regarded it as the general systemic antibiotic that it later proved to be. It must be remembered that Fleming was influenced by the prevailing views of his time, and during the early 1930s the concept of 'intravenous therapy', that is, that a bacteriocide could prove effective against bacterial infections when injected into the body, was widely discredited. There is also some evidence to suggest that Almroth Wright, who was the head of the Inoculation Department at St Mary's and Fleming's boss, discouraged Fleming from the view that penicillin might be a useful therapeutic agent. The strength of Wright's opposition was revealed by Fleming's friend and colleague V. D. Allison in 1979: 'Wright had been the reverse of enthusiastic about the curative value of penicillin when the manuscript of the first paper was submitted for publication. So much so, that he had demanded the omission of the short paragraph suggesting its employment for surface infections – meaning local infections.' Fortunately, Fleming stood his ground and the offending lines were included. However, it cannot have been easy for Fleming to maintain any kind of faith in penicillin in the face of the prevailing orthodoxy and, more obviously, of the criticism of his own boss, who was well known for his strong views and talent for critical argument.

Fleming's attempts to use crude penicillin involved the help of a friend, Arthur Dickson Wright, who was a surgeon at St Mary's and, like Fleming, a member of the Hospital's rifle shooting team. Working together, they used crude filtrates of *P. notatum* to try and achieve cures for infections like boils and long-standing leg ulcers. The results were promising but not spectacular. It seemed that whenever a suitable patient was found then no penicillin was available, and vice versa. As Fleming never found a method of storing, concentrating or purifying crude penicillin, it is perhaps not surprising that these clinical experiments were doomed to failure. Fleming was to achieve only one clear-cut cure using crude penicillin when, in 1932, he used it effectively to treat his laboratory assistant, K. B. Rogers, who had been suffering from a bad eye infection.

Although Fleming did a large number of laboratory experiments with penicillin, he never performed the apparently obvious animal experiment to show that his 'mould juice' could cure an artificially infected animal. However, anyone who has witnessed the foul-smelling product of fungal broth on meat broth medium will perhaps understand Fleming's reticence at the thought of injecting this brew into a living animal. It seems that the in vitro experiments which he performed convinced him that penicillin would not remain active in the body for long enough to kill the invading bacteria.

It was clear to anyone who handled these crude filtrates that penicillin would have to be purified before it could be used in medicine. Fleming's filtrates, in fact, contained remarkably little penicillin. There was no doubt that with his limited knowledge of chemistry Fleming would find it extremely difficult to extract the active ingredient from such meat broths. Fleming was not alone in being limited in this respect; like most bacteriologists of his generation, he had received only a rudimentary education in biochemistry. He was, however, well aware of these limitations, and so passed on the task of purifying penicillin to anyone who professed to having a superior chemical knowledge. As a result, some of the initial purification experiments were done by two young graduates, Frederick Ridley and Stuart R. Craddock. Ridley was training to be an ophthalmologist, while Craddock was a research scholar who had taken over from Pryce in Fleming's laboratory. It seems that Fleming gave these two young men only scant advice on how best to purify penicillin. In addition, they worked in cramped conditions and lacked the necessary equipment. Despite these problems they made remarkable progress.

The first thing Ridley and Craddock did was to grow up large quantities of penicillin on meat broth. They then set about extracting the active ingredient by, first, boiling the broth to reduce its volume. Unfortunately, this destroyed most of the penicillin, so next they attempted vacuum distillation, a process whereby a liquid is warmed in a flask held under vacuum, so that water, for example, can boil at relatively low temperatures. By using this method, the young men hoped to prevent the degradation of the heat-sensitive penicillin. However, they never achieved an efficient vacuum distillation with the primitive equipment which was available, the best they could achieve being a partial reduction of the crude product at a temperature of 40°C. This left them with a highly unpromising toffee-like mass which contained all of the broth impurities and only traces of penicillin. Further partial purification was then achieved by dissolving this mass in alcohol, ether or acetone.

It seems that Fleming received frequent written reports from Craddock about the progress of their work, so either he failed to fully understand what they were doing or was otherwise involved in what appeared more pressing work. The discovery that penicillin was soluble in solvents like alcohol was an important step forward, since it suggested a means by which partial purification might be achieved. While Ridley and Craddock's alcohol extracts of penicillin were potent, they were unstable, with most of the activity they contained being lost within a few days. The two young scientists then discovered that the stability of their penicillin extracts depended upon their pH. While the original broths were alkaline and unstable when vacuum distilled, the addition of acid to bring the pH to around 6.5 had the effect of allowing them to remain active for some weeks.

Fleming seems to have taken little direct part in these attempts to purify penicillin, although he does seem to have assayed the extracts produced by Ridley and Craddock to test for their antibacterial effects. It is not clear whether he used meat broth or more potent extracts when it came to treating infections.

Although Fleming appears to have given up on his attempts to use penicillin in medicine relatively soon after its discovery, there is little doubt that he never lost faith that it might one day be put to a therapeutic use. In 1931, for example, in a paper which he published in the *British Dental Journal*, he stated that 'Penicillin is valuable to us at present in the isolation of certain microbes, but it is quite likely that it, or a chemical of similar nature, will be used in the treatment of septic wounds.'

As we shall see in a later chapter, Fleming's initial views on the nature of penicillin changed dramatically during the early 1930s under the influence of a novel therapy called Besredka's antivirus. As a result, he began to believe that penicillin acted by influencing the patient's immunity, rather than by its direct effect in killing pathogenic bacteria. Such thoughts probably made him believe that the therapeutic properties of penicillin would be hard to demonstrate with the then rudimentary state of the science of immunology.

In 1934, one last attempt was made at St Mary's to purify penicillin. These studies involved a professional biochemist, Lewis B. Holt, who had joined the Inoculation Department to work with Fleming and Almroth Wright. Holt seems to have taken a completely individual approach to the problem of how best to purify penicillin. He began by extracting the meat broths containing penicillin with the solvent amyl acetate. After completing this step, he added sodium bicarbonate at pH 8 to the solvent and the penicillin moved from the solvent back into the aqueous phase to form a stable solution. Unfortunately, both he and Fleming appear to have missed the significance of this work: put simply, Holt had achieved the essential partial purification of penicillin as early as 1934.

Fleming and his colleagues were not the only people to take an interest in penicillin during the early 1930s. Another group of London scientists headed by Harold Raistrick also had a brief look at Fleming's new discovery. This work is particularly important since it demonstrates that the purification of penicillin was to be no easy task even in the hands of the world's foremost fungal biochemist. Harold Raistrick had been appointed as the first Professor of Biochemistry at the London School of Hygiene and Tropical Medicine in 1929. He had established a worldwide reputation as an expert in fungi and, in particular, the biochemical compounds which they produce when growing in culture. Raistrick's involvement in the penicillin story should therefore have provided the best opportunity for the early purification of penicillin to have been achieved.

It seems that it was W. W. C. Topley rather than Fleming who first alerted Raistrick's attention to penicillin. Fleming did not know Raistrick at the time. Bacteriologists, then as now, generally moved in different circles to mycologists.

Raistrick added penicillin to the selection of fungal products which his group were investigating. Assisting him were P. W. Clutterbuck, a biochemist, J. H. V. Charles, a mycologist, and a bacteriologist called Reginald Lovell. It was Lovell's job to test the antibacterial properties of the penicillin extracts obtained by the others in the team.

A culture of the penicillin-producing mould, still masquerading under the wrong name of *P. rubrum*, was obtained from Fleming. Both Raistrick and Charles questioned the accuracy of this identification, considering that the culture looked more like a strain of *Penicillium chrysogenum*. To settle the point, they forwarded a sample to the eminent US mycologist, Charles Thom, who was then the world's leading authority on the genus *Penicillium*. Thom pronounced the mould to be *Penicillium notatum*, despite the fact that the type culture of this fungus, that is, the culture used as a standard against which others can be identified, did not produce penicillin. This is an interesting anomaly since it means that only Fleming's strain was capable of producing penicillin, and anyone expecting to produce penicillin from a type culture of *P. notatum* would be disappointed.

With Fleming's mould correctly identified, Raistrick and his team began detailed investigations of its properties. Their brief was not to purify penicillin, but their experience should have pointed to the need to obtain the pure form so that it could be characterized with confidence. Raistrick already had a string of publications to his name detailing the properties of all kinds of obscure fungal by-products.

The first advance made by Raistrick's team was to show that *P. notatum* produced penicillin when grown on Czapek-Dox medium. As we have seen, this synthetic medium differs from the meat broths that Fleming had used to grow the fungus in being colourless and free from meat proteins. Next they confirmed that penicillin was soluble in various solvents. Then came the inevitable stumbling block – when an ether extract containing the active substance was evaporated to dryness, the penicillin it contained disappeared. Dumbfounded, Raistrick is quoted as having said: 'Such a thing was never known to chemists before. It was unbelievable; we could do nothing in the face of it, so we dropped it and went on with our investigations and experiments.' In particular, Raistrick's team now concentrated on the yellow pigment, called crysogenin, which is produced by *P. notatum*. Fungal pigments held some fascination for Raistrick so, unfortunately, the penicillin-producing mould by producing a pigment provided such an excellent opportunity for his attention to be distracted away from penicillin.

Clutterbuck and Lovell reported the results of their work at a meeting of the Biochemical Society, stating that 'a method of isolation of a crude, but highly active preparation has been evolved.' What exactly they meant by this is not clear. Masters, in his book *Miracle Drug* (p. 51), states that Raistrick did in fact achieve the all-important transfer from the ether extract of the culture filtrate to water, but was unable to produce penicillin in a stable, dry form. Unfortunately, the account of their work given at the Biochemical Society meeting gave the impression to anyone who was interested in purifying penicillin that there was no point in pursuing the task since it had already been achieved by a team led by one of the world's foremost fungal product chemists.

It seems to me that Raistrick and his team have been treated somewhat leniently by historians. While Fleming, the non-chemist, has been widely criticized for not having purified penicillin, these specialists have been exonerated. In the hands of an experienced fungal product chemist like Raistrick the task of purifying penicillin should have been relatively straightforward. However, it seems clear that Raistrick believed the task to be beyond the biochemical expertise available at the time. In his book *Antibiotic Producing Fungi*, published in 1963, the Russian mycologist, V. I. Bilai, confirms this view, stating: 'The eminent English biochemist, Professor Raistrick, stated at the Fifteenth International Congress of Physiologists in Leningrad in 1935 that he thought the production of penicillin for therapeutic purposes was almost impossible.'

One final irony concludes our look at Raistrick's brief sojourn with penicillin. Lovell, his bacteriologist, made a note to remind him to check the possibility that penicillin could cure an artificially infected mouse. In the event, like Fleming, he never performed this mouse protection test, and yet another early opportunity to develop the world's first antibiotic was missed.

Was Fleming the First Person to Discover Penicillin?

It is rare for a discovery to be made which has not been previously observed, or at least predicted. Although new ideas do, on occasion, arise from nowhere, most scientific breakthroughs are firmly based on earlier ideas and predictions. Penicillin, however, appears to be an exception to this rule. Prior to Fleming's work no one had suggested that certain fungi might produce a miraculous antibiotic. Had the thought occurred to earlier workers, then it is likely that they would have undertaken a screening programme in search of such a fungus. This is not to say that no one before Fleming had ever observed the antagonistic effect of micro-organisms, including fungi, on pathogenic bacteria. Indeed, some workers had even suggested that such antagonistic effects might find an application in medicine, while others actually went as far as to try and use the products of microbial metabolism to combat infection. However, no one seems to have suggested that a search of members of the genus *Penicillium* would yield a life-saving drug.

Despite this some medical historians have implied that Fleming was not the first to discover penicillin, and some have even suggested that his observations represent the last discovery of this antibiotic. However, only a few of the purported pre-Fleming discoveries of penicillin deserve close scrutiny, and by far the majority can be readily dismissed.

From the early days of microbiology many researchers noticed that certain microorganisms, both bacteria and fungi, could inhibit others when growing on culture media. Most of the early studies on this phenomenon were devoted to studies on bacterial, rather than fungal, antagonism. This work culminated in the observations by Emmerich and Low that *Bacillus pyocyaneus* was able to produce an antibacterial substance which they called pyocyanase. Pyocyanase will be looked at again in a later chapter. Although it had something of a chequered career, judging by the amount of interest shown in it, it must on occasions have been reasonably effective.

Many moulds can inhibit the growth of bacteria, including some which are pathogens. At first sight, the discovery of penicillin might appear to represent yet another example of the ability of a fungus merely to inhibit bacterial growth. Remember, however, that an experienced bacteriologist like Fleming, for whom examples of microbial antagonism would have been commonplace, was excited by his first sight of the penicillin effect. As we have seen, what caught his eye was not bacterial inhibition but bacterial lysis, and as far as we can tell, such lysis induced by fungi had not previously been reported.

Some interesting examples of microbial antagonism were detailed by Victorian scientists, some, like John Tyndall, who are better known for their studies in other branches of science. Tyndall was a mathematician and physicist by profession, but dabbled enthusiastically in the new science of microbiology.

It was scientific controversy which excited Tyndall's interest in the new subject. By the late 1870s two schools of thought existed concerning the origin of microorganisms and, for that matter, life in general. The first school, which in England was led by Charlton H. Bastian, championed the idea of spontaneous generation, and advocated the proposition that microorganisms arose *de novo* from the products of the culture medium. Their opponents, who included such notables as Louis Pasteur and Thomas Huxley, believed that microorganisms could only originate from other microorganisms. The impression is often given that the adherents of the spontaneous generation theory were somehow cranks. However, their arguments were well thought out and difficult to disprove, and had it not been for a well-fought, and often rearguard action from their opponents they might well have carried the day.

Some of Tyndall's experiments were directed towards demonstrating that the air is full of microbial spores which can contaminate nutrient solutions and germinate to produce new generations of fungi and bacteria. In an attempt to validate this hypothesis, Tyndall set up a large number of tubes containing boiled extracts of all manner of vegetables and meat, some of which, like snipe and venison, appear somewhat exotic today. These extracts were then exposed to the air over a period of a few weeks, during which time Tyndall meticulously observed the types of microorganisms which they supported. In his book *Floating Matter of the Air*, published in 1883, Tyndall describes what he observed in these infusions as follows: 'The mutton in the study gathered over it a thick blanket of *Penicillium*. On the 13th it had assumed a light brown colour, as if by a faint admixture of clay, but the infusion became transparent. The clay here was the slime of dormant or dead Bacteria, the cause of their quiescence being the blanket of *Penicillium*.' His observations are not restricted to the effect of fungi on bacteria. He notes that 'The Bacteria which manufacture a green pigment appear to be uniformly victorious in their fight with the *Penicillium*' and also 'The same absence of uniformity was manifested in the struggle for existence between the Bacteria and the *Penicillium*. In some tubes the former were triumphant; in other tubes of the same infusion the latter triumphed.'

I recently repeated some of these experiments, and to my surprise was able to almost exactly reproduce the same types of microbial contamination observed by Tyndall some one hundred years ago. Essentially four types of microbial contamination are usually seen in these exposed extracts. In some tubes, moulds grow alone, while others become cloudy due to the copious growth of bacteria. Nothing seems to grow in some of the extracts, while in others, both moulds and bacteria appear to grow together in harmony. However, without doubt the most interesting tubes, in relation to the question of microbial antagonism, are those which contain a surface plug of mould growing on an underlying clear extract covering a sediment of dead bacteria. Tyndall observed similar growth patterns to these, and explained the last type on the basis that the mould plug excludes air from the underlying bacteria, causing them to die. He was so taken with this explanation that he never performed the apparently obvious experiment of moving the mycelial plug to one side, to allow ingress of air, and then inoculating the clear liquid with a fresh supply of bacteria. Had he done this, he would have found that the bacteria do not grow despite having access to a supply of air. Quite clearly then, the fungus is producing some kind of material which is toxic to bacteria. Had Tyndall performed this experiment he might have gone on to suggest that such fungal toxins might be used in medicine to kill pathogenic bacteria. In the event, he was quite happy with his own explanation as to why the

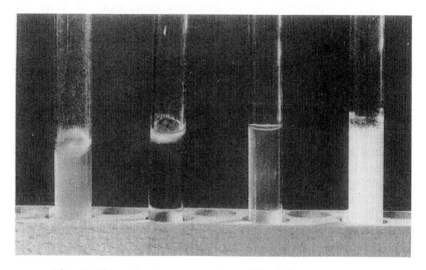

Plate 3 The author's reconstruction of Tyndall's experiment on
microbial antagonism. The all-important tube showing fungi inhibiting
bacterial growth is second from the left. (Photograph by the author,
© British Mycological Society)

bacteria died, and so missed the opportunity of doing further studies
which might have led to the discovery of a useful antibiotic.

Some historians regard Tyndall's work as an example of a pre-Fleming
discovery of penicillin. However, while Tyndall may have isolated a
penicillin-producing fungus, it is more likely that he isolated a mould
capable of producing an antibacterial agent which would have proved
toxic to humans and would have found no medical use whatsoever.
To demonstrate this likelihood, I again repeated Tyndall's experiments
and isolated one of the fungi which proved antagonistic to bacteria for
further study. This white mould produced a characteristic wine-red
pigment when growing on turnip extract, and was identified as
Verticillium psalliotae, a fungus which is a pathogen of mushrooms.
The red pigment turned out to be a compound called oosporein, which
although having antibacterial properties is also a mycotoxin, and is
therefore unlikely to find a use in medicine. These findings demonstrate
that even had Tyndall realized that his mould isolates were producing
an antibacterial agent, it does not follow that he would have discovered
penicillin; it is more than likely that, like me, he would have isolated a
fungus which produced a potentially toxic substance, rather than a life-
saving antibiotic. So while Tyndall's experiments helped defeat the

theory of spontaneous generation they can in no way be regarded as an early discovery of penicillin.

A number of other British Victorian scientists also observed examples of microbial antagonism, including William Roberts, Thomas Huxley and John Burdon Sanderson. During October 1870, Burdon Sanderson noted, for example, that bacteria were unable to grow in sterilized culture which had been contaminated with airborne *Penicillium*. Interestingly, his observations were made while he was working as Medical Officer for Health in the London Borough of Paddington, in which can be found St Mary's Hospital. The connection between Burdon Sanderson and Fleming's Hospital is further strengthened by the fact that Burdon Sanderson was appointed lecturer in Botany at St Mary's Medical School soon after it opened in 1854.

Observations on the ability of *Penicillium* species to inhibit bacteria were not restricted to Britain. In 1885, a New York surgeon called Frederick S. Dennis observed that *Penicillium glaucum* could 'annihilate bacteria', while ten years later, Vincenzo Tiberio of the Navy Hospital in Naples reported that an extract of a mould which he identified as *P. glaucum* prevented the growth of pathogenic bacteria. He then went on to detail how the extract could be used to treat infected rabbits, guinea pigs and rats. The Russians too can make reference to their 'penicillin pioneers'. These include the observations of Polotebnov and Manassein in 1872, on the inhibitory action exerted by 'green mould' on staphylococci and its therapeutic value in treating wounds. Other observations on the antibacterial activity of penicillia were apparently also made in Russia by Lebedinskii, in 1877, and Tartakovskii in 1904.

There is one startling example of how microbial antagonism was apparently put to therapeutic use some forty years before Fleming discovered penicillin. In 1884, a young girl living in Edinburgh was suffering from a wound which had been caused by a road accident. A variety of treatments were tried, but without success. Then the girl was given an experimental treatment which proved effective beyond all expectations. Obviously thankful for this minor miracle, the young girl asked the surgeon to write down the name of the curative substance in her personal notebook. The surgeon, who was none other than Joseph Lister, the father of antiseptic surgery, wrote down the word '*Penicillium*'.

Lister, then, seems to have used a mould extract to cure an infected wound, yet for some reason appears to have abandoned this successful therapy, and no further details of his methods have come down to us. Lister had observed the antibacterial properties of extracts of *P. glaucum* as early as 1871, and in the following year he wrote to his brother to say that 'Should a suitable case present, I shall endeavour to employ *P. glaucum* and observe if the growth of the organisms be inhibited in the human tissue.'

Why then do we not regard Lister as the discoverer of penicillin? Firstly, he seems never to have published details of his work, so we know nothing of the methods he employed, and secondly, he refers to the use of *P. glaucum*. This was a 'cover-all' term which was used by Victorian microbiologists to refer to any green species of *Penicillium*, or even of any green mould. The following eloquent description by Tyndall of the kinds of '*Penicillium*' which he observed in vegetable infusions clearly suggests that he at least was working with mixed cultures of fungi containing species other than *Penicillium*:

> The Penicillium was exquisitely beautiful. Its prevalent form was a circular patch made up of alternate zones of light and deep green. In some cases the liquid was covered by a single patch; in others there were three or four patches, each made up of its differently coloured zones. Reticulated patterns also occurred. Three kinds of Penicillium seemed struggling for existence, namely: – that just described; a second kind, of the same consistency and colour, but forming little rounded heaps instead of circles; thirdly, a wholly, voluminous, white mould, in the middle of which a zoned circle of the other mould sometimes formed an islet.

To say that the inhibitory effect of such mixed cultures of fungi on bacteria must be specifically due to the production of penicillin is clearly nonsense. We can never be certain which fungus Tyndall and Lister or their contemporaries actually employed in their studies. Many species of fungi produce penicillin, including around twenty different penicillia, and seven species of *Aspergillus*. On the other hand, fungi produce a wide variety of other antibacterial agents, some of which are toxic to humans. Modern fungal taxonomists believe that the term *P. glaucum* probably refers to a fungus called *Penicillium expansum*, which while it does not produce penicillin does produce an antibacterial agent called patulin. In a later chapter we will see that patulin was widely studied in the 1940s as a possible antibiotic and even as a curative for cancer. Unfortunately patulin turned out to be highly toxic and as a result has not found a use in medicine. It is quite likely, therefore, that Lister used an extract of patulin rather than penicillin to cure the infection of the girl he treated in 1884. Used in small quantities on a surface wound in this way patulin would have proved an effective antibacterial agent without being unduly toxic.

Perhaps the most impressive pre-Fleming studies on the ability of fungi to antagonize bacteria can be found in an unpublished doctoral thesis written by a Frenchman, Ernest Duchesne. Presented in 1897 to the Faculty of Medicine of the University of Lyon, this thesis describes studies which show that fungi are able to inhibit the growth of bacteria both in culture and when injected into an artificially infected animal. Duchesne concludes his thesis with the following statement, remarkable for its time: 'It can therefore be expected that the continued study of the facts of the biological competition between fungi and microbes, a study only outlined by us and concerning which we have no other claim than that of having brought here a very modest contribution, will lead, perhaps to the discovery of other facts directly useful and applicable to prophylactic hygiene and therapy.' Unfortunately, like Lister, Duchesne failed to publish the results of his studies. In 1907 he was called to army duty but was put on reserve because of ill health, and in 1912 he died at the early age of 38.

Other examples of the ability of fungi to inhibit bacterial growth were published throughout the early years of this century. In 1912, for example, Vaudramer showed that *Aspergillus fumigatus* could inhibit the tubercle bacillus, and he even claimed to have used it to cure some 200 tuberculosis sufferers! However, his results must have been very variable as his methods were never widely adopted. Then, in 1921, the German scientist Lieske observed the antibacterial properties of *Penicillium* culture extracts, but like many others before failed to realize the full potential of his observations.

So, by the time Fleming came to make his famous discovery in 1928, the situation regarding the origin of penicillin was quite straightforward – although there had been many previous reports of microbial antagonism together with an indication that fungal culture filtrates might cure infections, there is no real evidence to suggest that anyone other than Alexander Fleming discovered penicillin.

3

The Development of Penicillin

PENICILLIN'S FIRST DOCUMENTED CURES

Although, as we have seen, Fleming made a number of largely unpromising attempts to use crude penicillin to treat infected wounds, he was not to achieve the first effective cures with penicillin. This accolade fell to one of his former students, C. G. Paine.

When Cecil George Paine stepped down from the London train on to the platform of Sheffield's Midland Station and gazed across the bleak, smoke-filled city which would be his home for the next forty or so years, he could have had no idea that fate had chosen him to make a major contribution to the history of medicine, only to cruelly let him down. He had arrived in what was then the steel capital of the world to take up his first post as a newly qualified doctor. Although the scene which greeted him was bleak, it was no worse than the district around St Mary's Hospital, in Paddington, where he had been a medical student. After completing this initial training, Paine had accepted a conjoint post in Sheffield, that is, one which is shared, in this case between the Royal Infirmary and the University Medical School. Both posts together earned him £300 per annum. The Infirmary was a large, grim Victorian edifice situated about a mile from the University where Paine had been appointed Lecturer in Pathology.

Paine had first heard of penicillin while still a student at St Mary's, where he had attended Fleming's classes in bacteriology. After arriving in Sheffield he decided to use Fleming's 'mould juice' to try and cure patients, based on what he later described as a 'whim'.

Paine was born in London in 1905. He attended the Central Foundation School, and then Christ's Hospital School, where he stayed from the age of 11 until he was 19. There had been no medical tradition

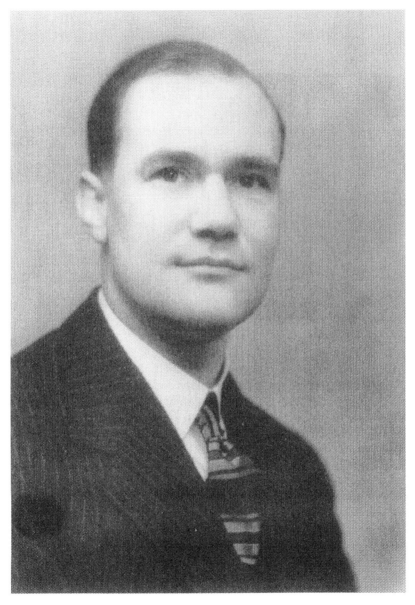

Plate 4 C. G. Paine in the mid-1930s, after he had become the first
person to achieve a cure with penicillin. (Courtesy of C. G. Paine,
© *Medical History*)

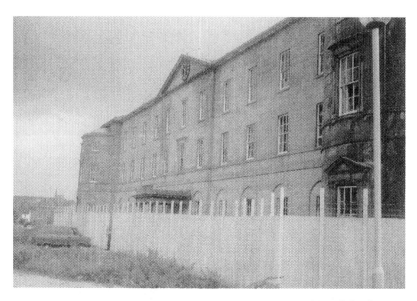

Plate 5 The Royal Infirmary, Sheffield, where Paine achieved the first
ever cure with penicillin. No longer a hospital, the building is now
undergoing extensive renovation. (Photograph by the author)

in Paine's family, but at school he excelled at chemistry although he
described himself as being 'an absolute dud at maths' – a fact which
appears to have had a major bearing on his decision to seek a career in
medicine. So in 1924, together with four of his schoolfriends, he
enrolled as a medical student at St Mary's. With his first MB already
gained while at school, Paine found the course relatively easy, and did
well enough to win the University Prize. He remembers being taught by
a number of 'giants of medical research' while at St Mary's, including
Sir Almroth Wright, Leonard Colebrook and, of course, Fleming.
Almroth Wright lectured to him on only one occasion, not, it turns out,
on a medical subject, but on logic! Colebrook taught him immunology,
apparently with great flair, while Fleming's lectures were devoted to
systematic bacteriology. Paine describes Fleming as being 'a shocking
lecturer, the worst you could possibly imagine', not because of any
inherent shyness, but because he never appeared enthusiastic about his
subject. Systematic bacteriology can hardly be described as the most
exciting subject in medicine, but the general opinion, not just Paine's,
seems to be that Fleming was a less than inspiring lecturer, a fact which
may help to explain why he failed to stimulate any enthusiasm for his
penicillin work amongst his contemporaries.

Paine and his student friends saw little of the research being done in the Inoculation Department at St Mary's, although they were encouraged to read 'the Orange Journal', the nickname for the journal which published Fleming's first penicillin paper. Paine even saw the original plate, but like most others who were given the privilege it failed to excite him as it had Fleming. Fleming's first penicillin paper was another matter, however, and when, at Sheffield, Paine was encouraged to initiate his own research programme he began by taking a look at the curative properties of crude penicillin.

Paine obtained a sample of the penicillin-producing mould from Fleming and grew it essentially as had been suggested in the first penicillin paper. He then tested it against a culture of *Staphylococcus albus*, to confirm that it could produce a potent antibacterial substance. Having obtained sufficient of the active crude penicillin, Paine decided to try it to cure patients suffering from infections caused by penicillin-sensitive bacteria. As he had no suitable patients of his own he had to enlist the help of the Hospital's dermatologist, Dr Rupert Hallam, who was also a pioneer of the medical use of radioactivity, and an ophthalmologist called Albert Nutt.

The first series of clinical tests with penicillin was done in collaboration with Hallam, and involved treating patients suffering from a skin infection called sycosis barbae. This infection of the hair follicle of the beard, caused by *Staphylococcus*, was quite common in pre-antibiotic days. Following infection, pus forms and the follicle becomes swollen and inflamed. The pathogenic bacteria lie deep in the follicle and as a result are difficult to reach and kill. Some experts recommended that the patient should avoid shaving, while others suggested that each individual whisker be removed, followed by the application of an equally painful dose of antiseptic! Paine's attempts to use penicillin to treat this infection involved soaking surgical gauze with the filtrates and then pressing them to the patient's face. The results of this treatment proved uniformly disappointing. Either the penicillin was too weak to prove effective, or perhaps more probably, it failed to reach the seat of the infection which lay deep in the hair follicle.

We can gain some clues as to why this work proved ineffective from the results of studies using crude penicillin on skin diseases during the early 1940s. Dr M. A. Cooke of the Royal Infirmary in Bradford, for example, cured cases of sycosis barbae using crude filtrates, but only after using daily sprays over a 6-week period. He also reported that in some cases there were relapses of apparent cures. Similar work by Taylor and Hughes also demonstrated the effectiveness of crude penicillin against this infection; however, these workers also noted the appearance of penicillin-resistant bacteria in cases of sycosis barbae. It is hardly surprising, then, that the short-term use of crude penicillin by Hallam and Paine should have proved so unsuccessful. Hallam, however, seems to have persisted with the view that microorganisms might be used to combat skin infections, since in 1932, in a paper devoted to the subject of recurrent boils, he describes how he applied yeast to their treatment. The following description of his treatment shows that it was as disappointing as the penicillin work had been: 'The yeast he [a Frenchman called Brocq] used may be different to the variety used by brewers in this country; certainly an extensive trial of the latter convinced me that it is useless for this purpose.' No mention is given in this paper of his attempts to use penicillin on skin infections.

Fortunately, Paine was not to be daunted by these early failures during his collaboration with Hallam. Instead, he decided to apply penicillin in the treatment of eye infections in collaboration with Nutt. These, he thought, would be ideal infections because the penicillin could easily reach and kill the invading bacteria. This time the treatments proved dramatically successful. The eye of one patient, a local miner, had been lacerated by a fragment of stone and had become badly infected. Tests conducted by Paine showed that the offending organism was a *Pneumococcus*, a dreaded pathogen whose presence would normally have necessitated the removal of the patient's eye. However, following irrigation with penicillin, the miner's eyesight was saved.

The next success achieved by Paine and Nutt involved a disease called ophthalmia neonatorum, an infection occurring in the eyes of babies which was relatively common in pre-antibiotic days and was responsible for much of the blindness in the newborn. The disease is particularly dangerous when the organism involved is the gonococcus (*Neisseria gonorrhoeae*), the cause of gonorrhoea. The infection was passed to the child from the mother during birth. It could to some extent be prevented, or even cured, by washing the eyes with a solution of silver nitrate, but often resulted in loss of eyesight.

While sparse details of the above work have been known for some time, it is only recently that it has been confirmed, following the discovery, by myself and Dr Harold T. Swan, of evidence which conclusively proves that Paine used penicillin to cure patients as early as 1930. This new evidence appears in the form of two case notes which refer to the use of penicillin by Paine and Nutt in two cases of ophthalmia neonatorum.

The first case note refers to the treatment of a 3-year old baby called Peter who was admitted to Mr Nutt's female ward on 28 August 1930. The baby is recorded as suffering from 'bilateral ophthalmia neonatorum of gonococcal origin, with copious discharge from the eyes'. Quite clearly, the baby had contracted gonorrhoea from its mother at

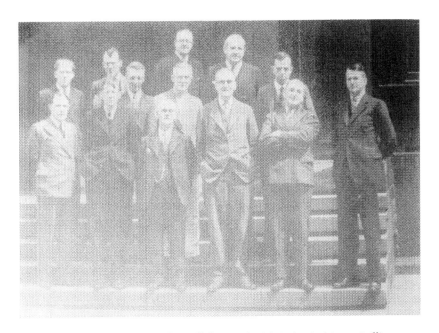

Plate 6 The surgeons who collaborated with Paine in his penicillin work. Taken in 1922–3, Rupert Hallam is standing on the front row (third from the right), while Albert Nutt is at the rear (second from the left). (© British Mycological Society)

birth. Peter had initially been treated in another Sheffield hospital at Nether Edge, but, after 3 months of conventional and unsuccessful treatment, he was transferred to the Royal Infirmary. On 25 November, Paine and Nutt irrigated the baby's eyes with a solution of crude penicillin. The treatment proved a complete success and Peter was allowed home on 11 December 1930.

This case was followed by a similar one, this time involving a baby girl called Sheila, who was only 6 days old when she was admitted. This time the eye infection was less specific, caused by what was termed 'diptheroids'. But once again the treatment was a complete success and, like Peter, Sheila was released from hospital in time to spend Christmas with her family.

An interesting feature of the first case note is that it contains the word 'Pinicillin', rather than penicillin, which suggests that the doctor or nurse who filled in the record was quite unfamiliar with the new substance.

The reader may be interested in learning how these case notes came to be discovered. In 1983 I re-read the account of Paine's work in

Masters's book *Miracle Drug* and wondered if there was any more to be discovered about Paine's apparently successful work. So I began enquiring about Dr Paine in the hope that perhaps he had left some unknown record of his work. It had generally been believed that Paine had done his penicillin work at the Jessop Hospital in Sheffield, so I began my enquiries there. At the outset of my researches I assumed that Dr Paine was dead, so when I eventually contacted his daughter, Mrs Elizabeth Joyce, I hopefully enquired if her father had left any notebooks that I might examine. To my complete surprise, she replied by suggesting that perhaps I should ask him myself! Dr Paine was very much alive and living in Devon. So, on Sunday 12 February 1984, I sped down the motorway, eager to meet the man whose life's work I had been somewhat ineffectively researching over the preceding months. I had been warned by one of Dr Paine's former students that he was something of a stern character, but I need not have worried. He turned out to be generous in his hospitality, and I soon learned that he was an accomplished amateur artist as well as an excellent cook!

Throughout the course of that afternoon, Dr Paine demonstrated his amazing memory for his Sheffield penicillin work, and included many details of which I was unaware. Unfortunately, he could only inform me that he had not kept any records of this work and as far as he was aware there were no case notes relating to it. So I returned to Sheffield with a more thorough knowledge of Paine's penicillin work, but no firm evidence to back up what was essentially only hearsay evidence that Paine had been the first person to achieve a cure with penicillin. However, quite by chance, someone recommended that I might contact Dr Harold Swan, a medical historian at Sheffield University who was involved in a study of the history of the old Royal Infirmary. Dr Swan had never heard of Paine, but to my amazement he told me that he was currently involved in checking through case notes at the Infirmary, with the brief of destroying the ones which were no longer of any use. Thrilled by this coincidence, I asked Dr Swan if he could search the notes for any reference to Paine, Nutt or Hallam. As I am not medically qualified, this laborious task fell entirely to Dr Swan. A few weeks later, he visited my office to inform me that he had found nothing, and that in any case it was like looking for the proverbial needle in a haystack. My obsession with the Paine story was such that I felt no compunction in asking him to have one more try! This he did, and within a week or so he returned, beaming, with two large photographs of the all-important case notes in his hand. Over the next few months Dr Swan and I gathered together all the information we had on the Sheffield penicillin story, and wrote a paper which was published in the journal *Medical*

History, from which details eventually found their way into the popular press.

In recognition of his pioneering work on penicillin, Dr Paine was later awarded the honorary degree of Doctor of Medicine by Sheffield University. Why then is Paine's name not more widely known as the first person to achieve a cure with penicillin? The main reason is that he never published any of the work, nor did he ever present it at a scientific meeting. Although Paine was a relatively young man he was already in the process of publishing work in the medical literature, yet he wrote not a word about his penicillin work. It seems that he thought he had insufficient hard data to warrant publication. While there was probably some truth in this view, a note from him on the work might have been accepted by a medical journal. Had even a brief description appeared in this way, then it might have alerted the medical world to the potential of penicillin. Such comments are, of course, made with the knowledge of hindsight, but it nevertheless remains something of an enigma as to why neither Paine nor Nutt made any public reference to their penicillin work. Both of them often gave short communications at local medical meetings held in Sheffield, yet they never said a word about penicillin!

Another surprising feature of the Paine story is that having achieved some remarkable cures he suddenly stopped working with penicillin and moved to another area of research. Crude penicillin's instability obviously played a part in this decision since, like Fleming, Paine never found a means of storing penicillin for use when it was needed. He also realized that he lacked the necessary chemical knowledge to attempt its purification. Later work was to confirm that the penicillin present in filtrates was reasonably unstable, losing all of its activity within two days at 37°C and after four to six days at room temperature.

Most importantly, however, just as Paine achieved his positive results with penicillin, he was offered a new post which involved promotion, a pay rise and, most importantly, the opportunity to work in an area of medicine which particularly fascinated him. The move took him from the urban grime of the Royal Infirmary to the Norton Annexe, a hospital set in pleasant parkland on the outskirts of Sheffield. Here Paine was to devote most of his career to the study of puerperal fever. Over the first six or so years of this work he concerned himself with studies on the subtle difference between different strains of bacteria which infected the womb, and how they were spread. It was during this period that he designed an efficient surgical mask which was marketed by Robinsons of Chesterfield under the trade name 'The Cestra Mask'.

Before commencing work at the Norton Annexe, Paine spent a few months working in London at the newly opened Queen Charlotte's Hospital, where he gained further experience of puerperal fever under the tuition of Leonard Colebrook and his sister Dora. At last Paine was in his element, devoting most of his time to a disease which so fascinated him, and for which a cure was so desperately needed. It is perhaps not surprising, therefore, that he dropped his somewhat speculative studies on penicillin therapy. Ironically, penicillin was to be dramatically successful in the treatment of puerperal sepsis, so it is possible that Paine might have achieved some cures had he irrigated the womb of infected women with his crude filtrates.

Dr Paine is, of course, fully aware of his missed opportunity. At the end of our interview I asked him where he placed himself in the penicillin story. His reply was one of great humility: 'Nowhere – a poor fool who didn't see the obvious when it was stuck in front of him. I suppose that there were many things that conspired to stop me doing it. I'm sorry but there it is. It might have come onto the world a little earlier if I'd have had any luck.'

Plate 7(a)

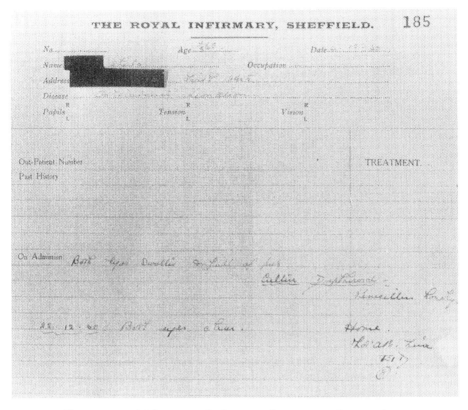

Plates 7(a) and 7(b) Recently discovered case notes showing the world's first cures using penicillin. (Courtesy of South Yorkshire County Archive, © *Medical History.*)

However, Paine can at least take heart that his work did have an influence on the history of penicillin and probably caused it to be used in medicine sooner than it otherwise might have been. In 1932 he discussed his work with the newly arrived Professor of Pathology at Sheffield University. This conversation took place in the quadrangle outside the room in which this book is being written. The Professor, to quote Paine, took 'not the slightest interest at that time'. Yet six years later he was to begin a programme of research which would lead to the purification of penicillin and its introduction into medicine. The Professor in question was, of course, Howard Florey who, with the help of Ernst Chain and other members of the Oxford team, would give penicillin to the world as the first of the 'wonder drug' antibiotics.

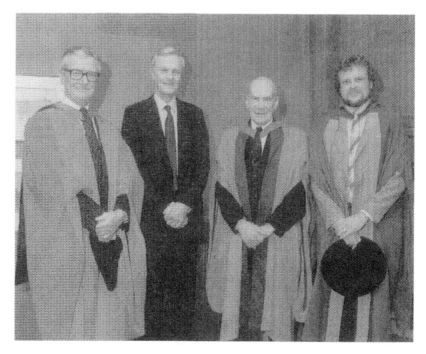

Plate 8 C. G. Paine receiving an honorary MD from Sheffield
University, March 1987. Paine is standing second from the right.
Also shown are the author (extreme right), Dr H. T. Swan and
Professor R. Richmond (extreme left). (© Sheffield University)

PENICILLIN: THE WILDERNESS YEARS

It is very unlikely that a medical practitioner working in the mid-1930s
would ever have heard of penicillin. Even a specialized bacteriologist
might have regarded it as something of an oddity which he might
occasionally have to prepare in order to selectively isolate certain
pathogenic bacteria. After Holt's attempt to purify penicillin in 1934,
little interest was apparently shown in Fleming's 'mould juice'. Why so
few medical scientists took an interest in penicillin is something of a
mystery. Ronald Hare, the late eminent bacteriologist and expert on the
history of penicillin, is, however, quoted as saying that the team
working on puerperal fever at Queen Charlotte's Hospital (which for a
short time included Paine) considered using penicillin, but never got
around to it.

The next development in the penicillin story takes us for the first time away from Britain and to the United States. Here, a young bacteriologist called Roger Reid read Fleming's paper and, while working at the Division of Bacteriology at the State College of Pennsylvania, added his own contribution to the then limited knowledge of penicillin.

After testing some 23 different moulds, Reid confirmed that penicillin production was not a widespread ability amongst fungi. He also concluded that penicillin was not bacteriolytic. In view of the lysis which had first attracted Fleming's eye this appears to be a contradictory finding. One can only conclude that the Fleming isolate quickly mutated after only a few transfers to fresh media, and somehow lost its ability to lyse bacteria on the way. As Reid was a research bacteriologist and had no patients of his own, he could do nothing to further penicillin's clinical use.

Charles Thom, the eminent US mycologist, remembered sending samples of Fleming's mould all over the United States during the 1930s, although after Reid's work nothing more was published on penicillin until 1940, when Dr S. Bornstein of the Beth Israel Hospital in New York published a paper describing an extension of its use in differential isolation media. This work appeared in the *Journal of Bacteriology*, whose editors received Bornstein's paper on 1 August 1939.

This small number of publications did not mean that no one was taking an interest in penicillin. For example, J. W. Fulton, of whom we will hear more later, made a search of the records of the Yale School of Medicine and found reference to the fact that in 1930 a scientist, who was not named but who apparently was later to become eminent, applied for funds to study the therapeutic potential of penicillin. Unfortunately the grant request was refused, doubtless because the work was thought to be of little practical use!

What of Fleming's commitment to penicillin during this period? There are a number of anecdotal references which suggest that, although he did no further work on penicillin after 1934, he was still convinced that it would one day find a place in medicine. For example, during that year, Fleming is said to have told a St Mary's doctor, G. L. M. McElligott, that penicillin might be useful in the treatment of venereal disease. McElligott described his discussion with Fleming as follows: 'I shall not forget the day in 1934 when he showed me the famous contaminated culture with the prophetic comment – "That stuff should be good for your patients" – and how the subsequent discussion on ways and means ended with his saying "it's up to the chemists now, I'm no chemist."' A similar recollection was made by another St Mary's doctor, A. G. Cross: 'Penicillin was on his mind all the time and in the minds of those who worked with him. I remember going up to his laboratory in the middle 1930s with a large carbuncle on the neck and one of his colleagues said, "If only Flem would make some more of that penicillin stuff we'd soon cure that neck." ' Ernst Baumler, in his book *In Search of the Magic Bullet*, also states that on leaving a lecture on Prontosil given in 1935 by Domagk, Fleming told Dr Douglas McLeod that he had something much better than Prontosil but nobody was interested, and that he could find no chemist who would take the trouble to isolate the substance for him.

There is evidence to suggest, however, that by the end of the 1930s, the major US pharmaceutical companies were beginning to take an interest in penicillin. In the autumn of 1940, for example, Merck, encouraged by Selman Waksman, produced some 9 litres of crude penicillin. By that time several other US pharmaceutical companies were taking an interest in penicillin. E. R. Squibb, for example, had made a survey of the penicillin literature as early as 1936, while other companies to show an interest included Eli Lilly, Lederle, Winthrop, Parke Davis and Upjohn.

Despite these isolated signs of interest, little work was done on penicillin after Fleming gave up trying to purify it and use it in the treatment of wound infections. It remained a laboratory curiosity, the product of one of Fleming's interesting but worthless observations. However, by 1940 the situation was about to change dramatically.

THE OXFORD GROUP

On 27 December 1940, while German bombs were raining down on London, a 43-year old policeman, Albert Alexander, was admitted to the Briscoe Ward of Oxford's Radcliffe Infirmary. He was close to death, suffering from an infection which had begun as an innocent scratch from a rose bush only a month before. Now pathogenic bacteria had invaded the tissues of his face reaching his eyes and scalp. He was given massive doses of a sulphonamide, but the wound continued to suppurate, and produce multiple abscesses all over his face and forehead. On 3 February his eye was removed, by which time the infection had reached his lung. Then, on the twelfth of the month, Dr Charles Fletcher gave him an injection of 200 milligrams of partially purified penicillin, followed by samples of half this dose at 3-hourly intervals. By the next day, the patient's temperature was normal and he could sit up in bed and take his meals. Penicillin was in such short supply that small quantities had to be extracted from the patient's urine, and then re-injected into his veins. Albert Alexander's condition continued to improve until, tragically, the supplies of penicillin ran out.

His condition deteriorated rapidly; his lungs became irreversibly infected and on 15 March he died. Penicillin had temporarily halted the infection in this desperately ill patient, but in the end it had failed. Perhaps the infection was just too well established, but in any case there was just too little penicillin available to overcome such a massive infection.

Purified penicillin had failed its first test, but successes were soon to follow. Its second trial involved the treatment of a 15-year old boy with an infected femur and a 48-year-old labourer with a huge carbuncle on his back. In both cases, penicillin proved a complete success. The carbuncle case was not as trivial as it might first appear, since the man was severely ill, with a high temperature and enlarged glands. Again, this case aptly illustrates how, prior to the appearance of penicillin, even the simplest of infections could cause severe illness and even death.

These first successes with penicillin contrast with some tragic failures. One case involved a 4-year old boy, who was admitted to the Collier Ward of the Radcliffe Infirmary under the care of Professor Witts in 1941. Following an attack of measles, the young boy had developed an infection in one of his eye sockets, from where it had travelled to the base of his skull. Sulphonamides were given without success, until on 13 May, penicillin treatment was begun. The boy was by now semi-comatose and there were signs that he had contracted meningitis. By the third day of the penicillin treatment his condition began to improve; the swelling in the eyes retreated and he was emerging from coma. The infection had been defeated, and the treatment was stopped so as to preserve the remaining supplies of penicillin. Then on 27 May, the boy had a sudden convulsion and he died four days later. The tragic outcome of this case was later shown to have been caused by a burst blood vessel in the boy's brain. Yet again, penicillin had shown its dramatic potential, but the patient had died.

The next case, however, would leave no one in any doubt that penicillin was capable of achieving miracles. A young boy had been admitted to the Rowney Ward of the Oxford Infirmary, under the care of Dr Cooke, on 6 May 1940. He was suffering from a bad case of osteomyelitis of the left femur. This infection, caused by staphylococci, was then relatively common amongst children. We shall see in a later chapter that in the 1930s, particularly in the United States, doctors were so desperate to find a cure for this infection that they even resorted to the use of live maggots to clean the wound! Now there was a much more acceptable and potentially far more effective treatment available in the form of purified penicillin.

The boy was initially given a 7-day course of sulphathiazole, but without success. Then the doctors drained his hip, an operation which did little to ease his intense pain, and he remained desperately ill. On the 6 June, penicillin began to be administered by continuous intravenous drip; if it failed the boy would almost certainly die. The miracle happened. By 9 June he was feeling much better, his temperature was normal and the pain in his hip had eased. Then, worryingly, his temperature began to rise intermittently or 'spike', raising fears that he might have an uncontrollable secondary infection. Fortunately, it turned out that these variations in body temperature were due to impurities in the penicillin.

Penicillin had saved the boy from certain death, but so serious had the infection been that he continued to suffer from a bad limp, and had to undergo intensive orthopaedic rehabilitation over the following two years. A letter sent to the Hospital in 1943 by the Oxford Education Committee enquiring about the boy's medical history provides an interesting sequel to this case. It seems that, now a teenager, he had tangled with the police and was about to be sent to an Approved School for correction – clearly, penicillin was not capable of achieving social as well as medical miracles!

These miraculous cures using purified penicillin were achieved during the early 1940s when, in the year from June 1940, some 100,000 civilians had been killed or seriously injured by German bombs. How was penicillin transformed from a laboratory curiosity to become a life saving drug at the beginning of the Second World War?

The fascist regime which was threatening the wholesale destruction of Britain's cities was, ironically enough, indirectly responsible for penicillin's rise from obscurity, since it was Nazi oppression that had forced a young German Jew, Ernst Boris Chain, to flee his homeland in 1933, and come to Britain, where he was to play a crucial role in the purification of penicillin. Chain was a brilliant young man whose prodigious musical talents almost directed him into a career as a concert pianist. Fortunately, he avoided this temptation and continued with his scientific career. Originally looking upon Britain as a temporary staging post on the way to Australia or Canada, events transpired to keep him in Britain. After a period as a research student in Gowland Hopkins's laboratory at Cambridge he moved on to Oxford to work with Professor Howard Florey. Florey, it will be remembered, had earlier been Professor of Pathology at Sheffield. An Australian by birth, he had established himself as one of Britain's premier medical researchers, who was particularly keen to wed together the two sciences of Pathology and Biochemistry. Florey had recently become interested in lysozyme, the first of Fleming's major discoveries. In Chain, he saw the perfect young man, who had the necessary knowledge of biochemistry to help him disentangle the secrets of lysozyme.

Chain soon concluded the lysozyme work and, by 1938, was looking for a new project to satisfy his immense talents. Florey suggested that perhaps he might wish to look at some of the other naturally occurring antibacterial agents. Accordingly, Chain began a search of the vast literature concerning these compounds. He eventually found reference to some 200 papers on microbial antagonism including, of course, the famous one by Fleming. He was interested in this paper because it appeared to provide an example of a fungal lysozyme. However, perhaps tired of lytic phenomena, he seems to have initially taken a particular liking to another antibacterial agent, called gramicidin. Florey, though, was keen that he concentrate on penicillin. Did Paine's work influence him in this decision? It would seem that it did. Although Florey is often portrayed as knowing little about penicillin before Chain 'stumbled' across Fleming's paper, this is certainly not the case. He had been on the editorial board of the journal which published Fleming's first penicillin paper and there is every likelihood that he may have helped in its editing. He also knew Fleming quite well and they frequently met at scientific meetings. Considering Fleming's obsession with his latest discovery, it is unlikely that they would have failed to have discussed penicillin. Finally, of course, Florey heard of penicillin's curative potential from Paine in 1932. He maintained that he had forgotten all about Paine's work by 1938, and that it in no way influenced his decision to choose penicillin for further study rather than one of the myriad of other antibacterial compounds available. However, one of his former students recently wrote to me to say that Florey mentioned Paine's work in an undergraduate lecture given in Oxford in 1936, so it would seem unlikely that he could have forgotten about it by the time Chain began the search of the literature which led him to penicillin.

Both Florey and Chain maintained that their decision to devote their efforts to penicillin were based on scientific interest rather than the desire to introduce a life-saving drug. Chain, for example, explained his motives thus:

> I became interested – immediately – in Fleming's paper, not because I hoped to discover a miraculous drug for the treatment of bacterial infection which for some reason had been overlooked, but because I thought it had great scientific interest. In fact, if I had been working at that time in aim-directed scientific surroundings, say in the laboratory of a pharmaceutical firm, it is my belief that I would never have obtained the agreement of my bosses to proceed with my project to work on penicillin.

Those politicians who wish to restrict apparently purely academic research in our universities should perhaps dwell on the significance of these words! However, while Chain may have been solely motivated by scientific interest, there is evidence to suggest that Florey was more single-minded in his approach, and from the outset had his eye on the therapeutic potential of penicillin. For example, a letter to the *Medical Journal of Australia*, written by a certain K. H. Heard, states that in 1938 Florey told Sir Hugh Cairns that he thought that a major war was imminent and he asked Cairns what he would like in the next war that he didn't have in the Great War. Cairns is said to have replied 'some means of controlling infection', to which Florey replied that that was the answer he had expected and that he had decided to make his personal war effort in that direction. He then said that his reading had led him to believe that Fleming's penicillin mould or some work on pyocyanase looked most promising. Cairns apparently suggested tossing a coin to decide which of the alternatives it should be, and chance favoured penicillin. It seems, therefore, that Florey did have penicillin's therapeutic potential in mind before Chain began the work which would eventually lead to its purification and then introduction into medicine.

Before Chain could repeat Fleming's experiments he needed to obtain a culture of the original strain of *Penicillium notatum*. By an amazing coincidence a subculture was already kept in Florey's Department at Oxford. Chain described how he had recalled seeing someone working with a mould:

> Something clicked in my mind, and there was this woman – Miss Campbell-Renton who worked for Professor Gardner across the corridor. I went at once to find her and ask her whether I had seen her carrying a petri dish with a mould culture along the corridor that separated our laboratories, and she said she had. I asked if she knew the strain of the mould and if, by any chance, it was *Penicillium notatum*. She looked surprised and then said 'yes' it was, and that she had been using it for some time in the bacteriology lab to separate unwanted bacteria from cultures of *B. influenza* which were not sensitive to penicillin. I was astounded by my luck in finding the very mould about which I had been reading, here in the same building, right under our very noses. I could hardly believe it was true. Miss Campbell-Renton agreed to give me a sample and told me that it had been obtained from Fleming by Professor Dreyer, Florey's predecessor, who had thought for a time that it might have some relationship to his

interest in bacteriophage – but that he had lost interest when
it was seen that it had nothing to do with the subject.

Chain was helped in the early stages of the penicillin work by an
American, L. A. Epstein, who had also worked with him on lysozyme.
Although it began slowly, by September 1939 the work had shown
sufficient promise for Florey to ask the Medical Research Council for a
grant of £100 to help them continue. Although the request was
successful, they were given a mere £25, a grant which was hardly
generous in the circumstances. Nevertheless, the work went ahead.
Chain was given the task of producing purified extracts, while Florey
would concentrate on the animal tests. Norman Heatley, another of
Gowland Hopkins's graduates, was employed to help Chain and to act
as the group's bacteriologist.

Heatley's contribution to the development of penicillin has been
surprisingly underplayed, yet he made a number of important contributions. For example, little progress would have been made with penicillin
had he not developed an accurate means of assaying the purified
extracts to determine their activity, a method which led to the
establishment of the Oxford Unit, a standard measure of penicillin
potency. More importantly, it was Heatley who suggested that
penicillin might be recovered from acidified solvent with alkaline buffer,
the method which, unknown to him, had been discovered by Holt in
1934. So it was Heatley, rather than Chain, who suggested the crucial
step which would lead to the successful purification of penicillin.

The first, largely impure preparations of purified penicillin were
yellow, prompting the press to baptize the new drug 'Yellow Magic'.
Pure penicillin, though, turned out to be white. The first extracts of
penicillin contained about 99 per cent impurities, and only 2 units of
activity, compared to the 18,000 units per milligram present in the pure
product. One of the many surprises of the penicillin story was that this
mass of impurities did not prove toxic when injected into animals and
then humans.

When the first samples of partially purified penicillin became available Florey was away from Oxford and Chain, excitable and impatient
as ever, decided to go ahead with some preliminary animal tests without
him. However, as Chain was not licensed to experiment on animals, he
asked a colleague, J. M. Barnes, to inject into two mice a millilitre of
solution containing 20 milligrams of penicillin. The mice survived
unharmed. Chain describes how Barnes became involved as follows:

> Before I went to Barnes I had come to Florey at least four
> times over a period of several weeks, with fractions I had

isolated, with the request to assay them and carry out toxicity tests. The last time I appeared in the laboratory with this request, Florey turned to Mrs Margaret Jennings saying, pointing to me, 'In one of my weak moments I promised this man to test his fractions and here he comes pestering me again.' After these humiliating remarks in front of others not involved in the project, it became clear to me that Florey was not really interested in penicillin and I decided to ask my friend Barnes to do the first preliminary experiments.

Whether Florey was merely joking is not clear. Perhaps Chain was, as usual, being quick to take offence. Nevertheless, the fact that he had asked Florey to do the tests on a number of occasions, without effect, suggests that the generally held view that Florey was enthusiastic about the penicillin project from its outset is wrong.

Florey, it seems, was not at all pleased to find that this vital toxicity test had been done in his absence. It may well be this event which first opened the rift between Florey and Chain which would continue to widen over the coming years. Chain maintained that Florey was not involved in the initial animal tests with penicillin, and it was only after they had proved to be a success that he took an interest. Of course, Florey was the busy head of the Department and so could probably find little time to become involved in the day to day running of experiments.

Penicillin began its first major test as a therapeutic agent in animals as British troops were scrambling off the beaches at Dunkirk. At 11 in the morning on 25 May 1940, Florey, assisted by his laboratory technician Kent, injected eight mice with a virulent strain of streptococci. Four mice were set aside as controls. The others were treated with penicillin: two with a single dose of 10mg and two with 5mg doses given at 2-hourly intervals. Heatley spent most of the early hours of the following morning observing the infected mice. He wrote in his diary, 'The controls [infected but untreated mice] look very sick but the treated animals seem very well. I stayed at the laboratory until 3.45 am, by which time all four of the control animals were dead. It really looks like penicillin may be of practical importance.'

Heatley returned to the laboratory at 11.45 am and found both penicillin-treated mice alive and well. Just after 1 pm that day Florey called a meeting where the results were excitedly discussed with Heatley and Chain. They decided that it would be necessary for Heatley to produce some 100 litres of crude penicillin a week if the work was to proceed with sufficient pace. Florey also realized that a full clinical trial of the new compound would be necessary if the pharmaceutical companies were to be persuaded to produce penicillin in bulk.

Florey's next step was to employ Edward Abraham to help Chain with the development of large-scale purification methods, and also to determine penicillin's structure as a prelude, they hoped, to its synthesis. One of the first breakthroughs in purification came in 1941, when Abraham and Chain employed the new technique of adsorption chromatography. This involved passing the unpurified penicillin down a column of alumina, on which the pure material was held while impurities passed through. The penicillin so retained could then be extracted from the column with the aid of solvents. From that point on penicillin was no longer a laboratory curiosity.

The Oxford team, urged on by Florey, did their utmost to produce sufficient penicillin for the first small-scale clinical tests. The work continued apace throughout the summer of 1940 when, in August, the Oxford team's first paper on penicillin appeared in the *Lancet*. One might imagine that this paper would have caused a clamour from the pharmaceutical industry, all keen to get involved in large-scale penicillin production. This was not the case, however. It seems that these companies were too much involved in the war effort to want to spend time and money in what was still a largely speculative project.

One person who was stimulated into action by the appearance of the *Lancet* paper was Fleming. An entry in one of Florey's small pocket diaries, held in the Florey Archive at the Royal Society in London, records the single word 'Fleming' for 2 September 1940. Fleming's arrival in Oxford, almost 12 years to the day since he had discovered penicillin, was, therefore, not the complete surprise which penicillin mythology suggests. Chain, however, was somewhat shocked to learn that Fleming was about to visit, because he had assumed that he must have long since been dead!

Fleming entered the Dunn Laboratory with the words, 'I've come to see what you've done with my old penicillin.' These apparently innocent words were to be interpreted by some as meaning that Fleming had come to establish priority for penicillin. This seems somewhat churlish in view of the fact that he had discovered penicillin and stayed loyal to its potential even in the face of total disinterest.

The initial relationship between Fleming and Florey was good to the point of being amiable. It would later turn sour, but there were no signs of this on that first visit. Fleming returned to St Mary's with a sample of the Oxford penicillin, and tested it to discover that it was far more potent than any of his own samples. A month later, he lectured to the Pharmaceutical Society on the subject of 'Antiseptics in Wartime Surgery', and for the first time in several years publicly mentioned penicillin. On the following day, 15 November, he again wrote to Florey, saying that he would forward a sample of the penicillin-producing mould which, because it produced less yellow pigment, might produce penicillin which could be more readily purified. He concluded his letter with this optimistic statement: 'It only remains for your chemical colleagues to purify the active ingredient and then synthesize it and the sulphonamides will be clearly beaten.'

Fleming was not the only scientist to respond to the appearance of the Oxford group's paper. Across the Atlantic, Dr M. H. Dawson of New York's Columbia University and Presbyterian Hospital, immediately recognized penicillin's potential and obtained a culture of Fleming's mould from Roger Reid. Together with Gladys Hobby and Karl Meyer, he began to produce sufficient penicillin to treat patients suffering from bacterial endocarditis. In this infection, bacteria become lodged in the heart valves end eventually destroy them, killing patients only a few months after they become infected. Unfortunately, the New York group were unable to produce enough penicillin to effectively demonstrate its worth in the treatment of this disease but, once again, its potential was clear enough.

Back in Oxford, Florey's laboratory had been transformed into a mini factory which was capable of producing some 500 litres of the crude filtrate, an amount which, after purification, was only sufficient to treat four or five patients! To achieve this level of production, Florey employed half a dozen 'penicillin girls', who were paid £2 a week to inoculate the flasks and then extract the crude penicillin. By the beginning of 1941, sufficient penicillin had been accumulated to begin the trials described at the beginning of this chapter. In 1942, a much bigger trial was set in motion, in which Florey's first wife, Ethel, played a leading role. In the meantime, Fleming had not been idle either. He had asked Florey to supply him with some penicillin so that he could treat an old friend, Harry Lambert, who was in a dangerous condition suffering from meningitis. Sulphonamides had been tried, but without success. Fleming decided that Harry's only hope was to receive penicillin intrathecally, that is, by injection into the spine. He phoned Florey to ask his advice. Florey could only reply that this approach had not been tried before, and that it would probably be very risky. Fleming nevertheless decided to go ahead and on 13 August 1940, he injected the Oxford penicillin into his friend's spine. The treatment proved a complete success and his friend made a remarkable recovery. Ironically, Florey had, at the same time, injected penicillin into the spines of artificially infected animals, with the result that they had all died! It was perhaps fortunate that Fleming did not hear of this news before he treated Harry Lambert, otherwise he would probably have hesitated and his friend would have died.

Fleming was so impressed by the effects of purified penicillin that he immediately made an appointment to see the Minister of Supply, who on the strength of this visit convened a meeting to discuss the possibilities of large-scale penicillin production. In this way, penicillin manufacture moved from small-scale laboratory production to factory production. The next phase of the story took place not in war-torn Britain but in the United States, where the Americans were to prove spectacularly successful in producing penicillin on a hitherto undreamt-of scale.

4

The Introduction of Penicillin into Medicine

PENICILLIN IN PRODUCTION

One of the enduring myths of the penicillin story is that soon after Florey's group purified penicillin the Americans stole it from the British. The British, who had been regarded as slow to develop penicillin, then had to suffer the indignity of paying royalties to the Americans on any penicillin that they produced.

The truth is that the British chemical companies made considerable efforts to produce large amounts of penicillin, work which involved a considerable degree of collaboration between companies who had traditionally been keen rivals. But primitive production methods and wartime bombing hampered these efforts. As we shall see, the production of penicillin on a scale sufficient to help win the war, and to be available soon after for civilian use, was largely the result of US expertise and commercial drive. The Americans certainly earned whatever they gained from their involvement in penicillin.

On 2 June 1941, Heatley met employees of ICI's Dyestuffs Division to discuss the possibility that they might wish to become involved in large scale penicillin production. The fact that these talks involved this section of ICI adequately demonstrates the minimal involvement which Britain's largest chemical company then had in the manufacture of pharmaceuticals. However, within a year and a half of this meeting, ICI were producing sizeable quantities of penicillin, and had made important advances in its manufacture. A production plant with an initial capacity of 500 litres of crude penicillin a week was set up at Trafford Park in Manchester. To achieve this ICI employed a rather dated process called shallow fermentation: Fleming's mould was grown in countless pint milk bottles, stacked in slanted rows to obtain the maximum degree of aeration. This primitive and space-consuming approach to penicillin production lingered on until 1947, when ICI moved over to the more efficient deep fermentation process.

During shallow fermentation, the penicillin-producing mould is grown on the surface of a shallow layer of nutrient medium, into which it secretes penicillin. The process was originally carried out in milk bottles and bedpan-like vessels, although later production methods involved the use of large trays incubated in a sterile room, much in the same way that some companies still produce citric acid. Initially, the entire UK production of penicillin used shallow fermentation methods. A London firm, Kemball-Bishop, who were experienced in the manufacture of citric acid by shallow fermentation, was busy producing relatively large amounts of penicillin using the tray method as early as 1942. By the following year, they were producing penicillin in metal milk churns, which were then sent up to Oxford for their contents to be processed.

The production of penicillin by deep fermentation methods involves growing a special strain of the fungus deep in the nutrient medium, which is continually stirred and aerated. The main advantage of this technique is one of scale, since vast quantities of crude penicillin can be produced without the continual need for small containers to be washed, sterilized, filled with medium, and then inoculated with the fungus.

Some idea of the rapid development which took place in penicillin production in Britain during this early period can be gained from the fact that Glaxo, who in December 1942 were producing just over 1,000 units of penicillin, had increased this amount some 25 fold by the following year and were producing a staggering 40 billion units of penicillin by January 1945!

By the mid-1940s, developments in the States had made surface culture production methods obsolete and from then on deep fermentation was clearly in the ascendancy.

THE ENTRY OF THE AMERICANS

It was obvious to Florey that the best hope for large scale penicillin production lay not in Britain, whose industry was being frequently disrupted by enemy bombing, but with the giant US pharmaceutical industry. So from the earliest days of the Oxford penicillin work, Florey had decided to seek US help. Florey was also worried about the prospect of an imminent German invasion during the early period of the Oxford penicillin work – so worried, in fact, that he and some of his colleagues smeared spores of the penicillin-producing fungus inside the linings of their coats – just in case the Germans might invade, making necessary the destruction of all the cultures and notes on penicillin production. Incidentally, early in 1944 the Nazi propaganda machine laid claim to the discovery of penicillin, a claim which they hoped would be strengthened by the award of the iron cross, first class, to Hitler's personal physician, Dr Theodor Morell. Needless to say, the Germans never managed to produce penicillin, except in trace quantities, and this award was in no way justified.

Florey was assisted in the task of seeking US help by an old friend and fellow Rhodes Scholar, John Fulton. Fulton records that on 3 July 1941, to his surprise, Florey and Norman Heatley arrived unannounced on his doorstep in New Haven. The two Oxford scientists had crossed the Atlantic by the luxurious clipper service, flying via Lisbon where they had had the opportunity to enjoy the delights of a neutral capital city in wartime. Florey had more than one good reason to visit Fulton: it gave him the opportunity to see his children, Paquita and Charles, who were evacuees and in the care of the Fultons for the war's duration.

Fulton wasted no time. He immediately introduced Florey to Ross G. Harrison, the Chairman of the National Research Council. Harrison suggested that they should first of all visit the eminent US mycologist, Charles Thom. It was Thom who, it will be remembered, had correctly identified Fleming's mould as *P. notatum*. Thom, in his turn, passed the British scientists onto Percy A. Wells, the Director of the US Department of Agriculture's Research Service.

Wells had been given the task of developing new uses for farm products, notably wastes. To promote this programme the USDA had recently opened the Northern Regional Research Laboratory in Peoria, Illinois. Here the Department of Agriculture's scientists had become particularly well known for their work on mass-producing the products of fungal fermentations. They were therefore in an ideal position to take on the penicillin work.

Florey and Heatley arrived in the small Midwestern town of Peoria on Monday 14 July 1941. Florey's visit was short, as he was needed back in Britain, but Heatley was to stay at Peoria until late November. Before he left, Florey managed to get the Americans to promise to let him have a kilo of the first penicillin to be produced there, so that he could begin that all-important full clinical trial. Heatley, meanwhile, passed on all the secrets of penicillin production to the US team.

One member of the Peoria team, A. J. Moyer, played a leading role in scaling up penicillin production when he discovered that yields could be dramatically improved by the addition of cornsteep liquor to the growth medium. This plentiful by-product of maize production was one of the waste products for which a use was being eagerly sought at Peoria. Moyer was something of a shadowy figure who was later to take out valuable patents in his own name on some of the developments which resulted from the penicillin research programme.

The Peoria scientists were to make two other major contributions to large scale penicillin production. The first was the recognition that economic production could be best achieved using deep fermentation, for which they would have to isolate, or otherwise develop, a new strain of Fleming's mould. Both of these aims were to be achieved when a strain of *P. chrysogenum* was isolated from a mouldy cantaloupe melon found by a Peoria woman, Miss Mary Hunt. She had earned for herself the nickname of 'mouldy Mary', because of her enthusiasm for finding new moulds which were then tested for their penicillin producing powers.

The next important American development was the use of mutagens, like X-rays, to produce new 'super strains' of penicillin producers. For example, an early mutant of the Mary Hunt cantaloupe strain yielded nearly 1,000 penicillin units per millilitre.

In 1943, the production of penicillin was given highest production priority, second only to the atom bomb programme. By 1944, the cost of treating a single severe bacterial infection with penicillin was $200, a figure which fell so rapidly that eventually penicillin would cost less to produce than did the packaging which contained it!

One winter morning, Robert Coghill, Head of the Fermentation Division at Peoria, visited Pfizer's penicillin production plant in Brooklyn and stood before the giant fermentation tanks, each capable of producing 10,000 gallons of crude broth. His words perfectly sum up the battle that had been fought and won for penicillin: 'I stood at the end of the production line and saw 100,000 unit vials of penicillin coming off quicker than I could count them. It was then that I knew that the battle had been won and that victory was ours. It had been a long road from Fleming's petri dish to the finished vials, ready for the physicians' hands.'

DID THE AMERICANS STEAL PENICILLIN?

In Britain, at least, the view is often expressed that penicillin was stolen by the unscrupulous Americans, a view which is almost as much a part of British folklore as is the notion that the US entered both World Wars at the point when they had already been won! It has frequently been pointed out that the British had to pay the Americans huge amounts of money in royalties for the privilege of producing what was, after all, a British discovery – even if it did involve the efforts of an expatriate Australian and refugee German!

The apparent failure of the British to profit from penicillin has often been cited as a perfect example of how we are supreme at discovery, but backward when it comes to marketing our discoveries and inventions. While there is some truth in this, two points must be borne in mind in relation to the industrial development of penicillin. The first is that penicillin, being a natural product, was, both at the time of its discovery and during its later development, not patentable. As a result neither Fleming nor the Oxford group could have taken out patents on penicillin, even in the unlikely event that they had considered it ethical to do so. Chain, however, perhaps because he was not influenced by the Hippocratic Oath, took a different view. He saw no reason why medical scientists should not profit from their discoveries. While few would argue with this view today, this certainly was not the case before the last war. Cecil Paine, for example, took it as something of an insult when I asked him if he would have considered patenting penicillin had he purified it.

The Americans, on the other hand, took a less idealistic approach to this question, and while penicillin itself could not be patented, they saw no reason why the production methods for which they had worked so long and hard should avoid this protection. What galled Florey and his team was that, having freely handed over their expertise on penicillin to the Americans, they found that some, like Moyer, took out foreign patents on their own work, and profited from them. For example, on 31 May 1945, Moyer's agents lodged three patent applications in the Patent Office in London where they received the numbers, 13674–6. Moyer's first British application was for culturing *P. notatum* in eight different ways, including deep fermentation. His second application claimed patents for 39 separate media, including many in combination with corn steep liquor. Not surprisingly, the British were annoyed to hear of these patents. On balance, however, it seems that the production agreements between the US and the British pharmaceutical companies were eminently fair, and there is little that we in this country need to grouse about.

Unquestionably, the outstanding difference between the American and British approach to penicillin development was the willingness of the US companies to employ the help of the Land Grant Universities, and to share their expertise in fermentation technology. Fortunately, the British pharmaceutical industry was quick to learn from the penicillin experience. As a result, they devoted more of their profits to in-house research and development, and made sure that later British developments in the field of antibiotic research were well covered by patents.

Penicillin: War Wounds to Wonder Drug

During the First World War, 150 out of every 1,000 battle casualties died of infected wounds. While the appearance of the sulphonamides had a dramatic impact on battle casualty mortality in the opening years of the Second World War, penicillin was to have an even more miraculous effect, such that from D-day to the collapse of Germany the death rate as the result of infected wounds amongst Allied soldiers was reduced almost to zero! Open fractures showed a recovery rate of 94 to 100 per cent, and penicillin meant that for the first time in the history of warfare, soldiers with burns of one fifth or less of their body surface made almost complete recoveries.

Although the Germans were well aware that the Allies had penicillin they never succeeded in producing it on a large scale, a fact which was a major contributory factor in their final defeat. There was some debate as to the legality of preventing penicillin-producing culture from reaching the enemy, since it could be argued that in International Law it was illegal to distinguish between friendly and enemy wounded. Despite this, the military potential of the new drug was fully recognized and, perhaps not surprisingly, cultures of Fleming's mould were not dispatched to Nazi scientists and doctors.

The first, inauspicious use of purified penicillin in a war zone took place on 17 August 1942, when it was used by Major R. J. Pulvertaft at the 15th Scottish General Hospital in Cairo. An obituary published in the *Daily Telegraph* of 16 June 1977 states that the first soldier to be treated with penicillin was W. J. McGowan. The obituary reads:

> First Soldier Treated with Penicillin – Mr William Johnston McGowan, who has died aged 67, was the younger son of the first Lord McGowan and the first Allied soldier to be treated with penicillin during the Second World War. While serving with the Sherwood Rangers he was wounded at El Alamein in October, 1942. The wound severed his sciatic nerve and turned septic bringing him near to death. At the time, ICI, of which his father was the Chairman, had almost completed experiments with the new drug. It was decided to make the first 'field test' on the chairman's son.

The accuracy of the dates given here is questionable since they disagree with those given in the following letter to Florey, written by Lord McGowan, dated 30 June 1943:

I think you will be interested in the following. One of my boys was seriously wounded about two months ago, a bullet from a German sniper entering his calf, going through the knee and out of the thigh. He was eventually taken down to Base Hospital at Cairo and for some little time the wound made progress. Subsequently however, septicaemia set in, and for a month he was on the 'dangerously ill' list. On the 9th of June, to be precise, a serious operation was performed on a large abscess near the heart. Fortunately I was able to have flown out a supply of penicillin for internal use, which arrived the day before the operation, and I am sure now that the doctors think that the use of penicillin was contributory in preventing death during the operation. For this, of course, I am grateful, and I want to extend my gratitude to you for all the work you have done on this drug, which has now made for itself a very great reputation.

A particularly interesting feature of this letter is, of course, that Florey did not know of, nor was he a party to, the decision to use penicillin in this way.

As we shall learn in the next section, Pulvertaft had been treating soldiers for some time using crude penicillin filtrates, but this was the first time that he had obtained access to the infinitely superior Oxford product. He decided to use his meagre supplies of the pure product to treat surface wounds. The first thing he noticed following its use was a reduction in the all-pervading smell of infected wounds. From now on, penicillin meant that surgeons would no longer be greeted with the foul smell of gangrenous wounds as they entered their surgical wards.

Florey gave the US forces' doctors their first experience of penicillin in 1942, when he collaborated with Lieutenant Colonel Rudolph Schullinger, who had arrived in Britain with the 2nd US General Hospital. Schullinger visited the RAF hospital at Halton and witnessed at first hand the dramatic effects of penicillin on badly burned fighter pilots. Despite writing numerous glowing reports to his superiors back in the States, Schullinger's pleas for further supplies of penicillin were largely ignored. Eventually, in May 1943, he received some 18 million units, which came with strict instructions that they were to be used only on US military personnel. To his credit, however, Schullinger released some of the penicillin for civilian use, and the life of a man in Shaftesbury Hospital was saved by five million precious units. The US Lieutenant Colonel was then invited to Oxford to see the production line, where Florey's wife Ethel had joined the team and was doing impressive work during a new series of penicillin trials. Ethel Florey's contribution to the clinical testing of penicillin has been largely overlooked. There is a charming story of how she would bicycle each day collecting bottles of urine obtained from penicillin-treated patients, from which the valuable drug was extracted. This tour of the local Oxford hospitals was known to the more sophisticated as 'the morning milk round', but, perhaps inevitably, it was more generally known as the 'P-patrol'!

During mid-May of 1943, Florey decided that it was time for him to see for himself what penicillin was achieving in the battle arena. He arrived in North Africa with Dr Hugh Cairns, and with the invasion of Italy, the tide of the war gave them a perfect opportunity to witness the effective use of penicillin on battle casualties. It was in North Africa that penicillin's effectiveness in treating gonorrhea led to the most noted controversy concerning its use in the war. General Poole, Director of Pathology at the War Office, described his dilemma to Florey in the following words: 'Was it better to restore invalids suffering from VD to the battlefield by using penicillin, or to reserve it for the longer term treatment of battle casualties?' Florey and Cairns replied that they favoured the latter alternative, because they perhaps rightly believed that the general public would not approve of the scarce supplies of the new wonder drug being reserved for men who had been enjoying 'the spoils of war', thereby leaving battle casualties untreated.

Poole, unable to resolve the dilemma himself, asked Churchill's opinion. In a classic non-committal statement, Churchill replied: 'This valuable drug must on no account be wasted. It must be put to the best military use.' Poole interpreted this, no doubt as it was expected he should, to mean that penicillin should be used to return men as quickly as possible to their units, which of course meant reserving it for VD cases!

By 1944, Allied supplies of penicillin were officially described as being 'unlimited'. Instructions for its use on D-day were published on 15 May 1944, some four years since Florey had walked across the University Parks in Oxford to see how the first mouse test had fared. In those four years, the production of penicillin had progressed from a minute trace to a limitless supply, a feat which was indeed the second miracle of the penicillin story.

THE RETURN OF CRUDE PENICILLIN

The large-scale production of the purified product should have relegated crude penicillin, that is culture filtrates of *P. notatum*, to merely an historical curiosity. However, crude penicillin made a surprising comeback into the medicine of the early 1940s. The reason for this is quite simple: despite the immense efforts of the pharmaceutical companies to produce purified penicillin, there simply was not enough to meet the ever-growing demand, since, as we have seen, what was produced was reserved for military use.

This supply problem produced a tragic situation. Doctors were aware of a treatment which they could not use. Florey was inundated with requests for a small sample of penicillin – just enough to save a child's life, for example. But he could do nothing; even special pleading from members of the government on behalf of doctors was to no avail. So while family practitioners and hospital doctors read with increasing frustration of this new wonder cure they were in no position to obtain supplies to help treat their patients. Faced with this dilemma, they either let their patients suffer or die, knowing that a cure was available, or else they took steps to manufacture their own penicillin. The production of pure penicillin was clearly well outside the expertise of the family doctor, and would prove difficult enough even for a hospital laboratory. Crude penicillin, on the other hand, appeared far less daunting to produce.

As we have seen, crude penicillin had been shown by Fleming and Dickson Wright to be useful in treating bacterial infections as early as 1929, while Paine achieved the first documented cure with Fleming's 'mould juice' in the following year. While a large number of remarkable cures were to be achieved in the early 1940s using crude penicillin, fears about its uncontrolled use dramatically limited its use. In any case, by the middle of the decade, large amounts of the purified product had become available, and 'homemade penicillin' was no longer needed.

The term 'homemade penicillin' gave the product a bad image from the start, since it implied that penicillin was being produced in an uncontrolled way in someone's kitchen. The popular press at the time made matters worse by giving the impression that any green fungus, obtained from mouldy bread or jam, was capable of producing penicillin. The *News Chronicle* of 12 November 1943, for example, boasted the headline' Penicillin made for 3d in kitchen'. Such irresponsible reporting forced the experts to reject, out of hand, the idea of using crude penicillin. They feared that people might unknowingly use a strain of fungus which produced a mycotoxin. For example, the *Sunday Chronicle* of 19 November 1943 reported an unnamed British authority who warned that 'It is absolutely essential to purify the drug. Crude penicillin might be made cheaply but it would be likely to contain deadly dangerous bacteria.' In fact, most of the crude penicillin used in this period was produced by scientists or hospital laboratory technicians, who had a good knowledge of microbial technique, and as a result the bulk of the supplies were produced under highly controlled laboratory conditions. By spreading unfounded fears about the use of crude penicillin the authorities unfortunately severely limited the use of this potentially life-saving substance.

Essentially three different approaches were taken to the use of crude penicillin to treat infections. In the first, filtrates of *P. notatum*, produced on a synthetic medium, were used to saturate an absorbent gauze, which was then applied to the infection. In a variation of this approach, the wound was directly irrigated with the culture filtrate. A second approach was to apply living mould to the infection, while, finally, filtrates of *P. notatum* could be added to agar, which was then forced deep into the wound.

A number of subtle variations on these techniques were tried, and most workers had their own favourite recipes or modes of application. One of the most interesting of these variations was described by two doctors of the Allegheny General Hospital in Pittsburgh, George H. Robinson and James E. Wallace. These workers actually grew a culture of *P. notatum* on gauze which was then transferred to the wound where it continued to grow and actively secrete penicillin. This approach was further developed by Julius A. Vogel, plant doctor of the Jones and Laughlin Steel Corporation in Pittsburgh. The success of this approach probably relies on the fact that penicillin-producing moulds excrete tiny globules of concentrated penicillin from the colony surface. An interesting connection exists between Vogel's methods and the mould therapy employed by James Twomey, which will be discussed in a later chapter, since in some studies, Vogel grew his mould on cornflour before smearing it on gauze and then applying it to wounds. In a similar way, Twomey grew mould contaminants on a starch mix which he then used to cure the skin infection, impetigo.

Without doubt, the most convincing use of crude penicillin in therapy took place on the island of Hawaii during the early 1940s. About 100 doctors on the Island were eventually to use the crude product, with what was described as 'outstanding success'. The filtrates were cheap to make and easy to transport, and proved to be remarkably effective against a wide spectrum of infections. The Hawaiian team concluded that: 'We feel now that a source of a rather scarce and potent drug is readily available to anyone who may be willing to produce it wherever he may be.'

While the Hawaiian experience provided the most systematic and thorough studies on the production and application of crude penicillin in medicine, by far the most dramatic use of Fleming's 'mould juice' came on 2 December 1942 when large quantities were used to treat burns patients in the notorious Coconut Grove Fire. On the night of 28

November, this Boston nightclub caught fire, resulting in the death of over 500 people. Fifty litres of penicillin, presumably in the crude form, were rushed with a motorcycle escort from the Merck factory in Rahway, New Jersey, arriving in Boston at three in the morning. By the following month, all second-degree burns victims who had received the penicillin had been released from hospital while the third-degree burns patients were progressing well.

The war in the Western Desert provided an excellent opportunity to demonstrate the value of crude penicillin. This work was done by R. J. V. Pulvertaft, who, it will be remembered, was one of the first war surgeons to have the privilege of using the Oxford penicillin. Pulvertaft, unlike the penicillin pioneers, had no shortage of suitable patients on which to try crude penicillin. Battle sepsis was rife in this theatre of the war, and many of the wounds proved unresponsive to sulphonamide treatment. Pulvertaft obtained a culture of Fleming's mould from a friend who was working for the pharmaceutical company of Burroughs-Wellcome, who were then exploring the possibility of penicillin production. Pulvertaft obtained no official backing for his crude penicillin work: in fact it is likely that his superiors would have reprimanded him had they known about it!

Pulvertaft's crude penicillin was produced in the cellars of the Citadel, one of the few places in Cairo which was cool enough to allow the mould to grow and excrete penicillin. He achieved a large number of cures with this product, and his papers are full of statements such as 'No discharge, wound healing', or 'No discharge, regaining feeling in hip'. Some of Pulvertaft's original reports have recently been unearthed by Dr H. V. Wyatt of the Department of Community Medicine of Leeds University. One report, dated the end of June 1943, is particularly interesting since it states that 'The crude product, applied externally to wounds, appears to be just as efficient as the purified product'; and also 'It has been injected intravenously into man in a dose of 200 cc without any reaction.'

Florey was apparently annoyed when he heard of Pulvertaft's work regarding it as 'an unnecessary and retrograde step'. Fleming, however, encouraged this work; it confirmed that his 'mould juice' could achieve cures without being purified. This fact no doubt had an important bearing on his attitude to his discovery of penicillin, since it meant that he need not regard his position as being subservient to the work of the Oxford group. It is interesting that when I interviewed Pulvertaft he consistently referred to Florey's 'concentrated penicillin'. As far as he was concerned, crude penicillin was itself a remarkable curative; in his view all that Florey's group did was to *concentrate* it.

Florey, on the other hand, probably felt that crude penicillin might tarnish the image of the purified product at a critical stage in its development. His views on the value of crude penicillin are given clearly in the following reply to a letter from a Dr J. F. Heggie, who wrote for advice on the production of the crude material in September 1942:

> In answer to your letter I would say this: that the manufacture of penicillin is not easy and I doubt whether a 'well equipped laboratory' is of much help. Fleming, for example, who has a well equipped laboratory, having seen the scale on which we had to work here, decided not to do anything about making penicillin. I do not feel that it is much help to use a solution of penicillin. Even if you made a little penicillin you would have immense difficulties of assaying, having a standard preparation etc. I would suggest that it would be better to wait until you can obtain penicillin from a manufacturer.

Florey's fears about the uncontrolled use of crude penicillin appear well founded, since supplies of dubious composition were sold on the Egyptian black market during the early years of the war. Pulvertaft himself related to me a story about how one of his sergeants sold the crude product, together with completely useless variants, to the highest bidder, even making sales trips as far as Syria and Trans-Jordan. Pulvertaft was to receive a number of complaints from other surgical centres that his crude penicillin was useless, complaints which no doubt reflect the activity of this renegade sergeant!

In the spring of 1944, newspapers in Britain revealed yet another experimental use of a crude penicillin preparation, this time called 'Vivicillin'. Headlines such as 'Secret of New Drug is Out – Vivicillin Saved A Lost Life – Plenty For All,' and 'Doctor as Guinea Pig – Tested New Drug on Himself' were blazed across the *Daily Mail* and *Sunday Dispatch*. The reports behind the headlines then went on to describe how the life of a 9-year old boy, Anthony Phillips, of Chesterfield Road in the London suburb of Barnet was saved by injections of Vivicillin. The lad was suffering from peritonitis which had developed from an infected appendix. Doctors dared not operate because the boy suffered from haemophilia, and an operation would have proved almost certain death. After Vivicillin treatment, the boy made what was called a 'miraculous recovery'. Vivicillin was first produced by Mr W. K. S. Wallersteiner, a biochemist, and Dr Hans Enoch, of the International Serum Company, both refugees from Hitlerite oppression. Vivicillin received its name because it contained penicillin in the living form. After some quite extensive animal trials, Vivicillin was first used at Wellhouse

Hospital, where the Medical Superintendent, Dr H. Roland Segar, was a close friend of Wallersteiner and Enoch. It seems that Vivicillin was 'a suspension of macerated *P. notatum* hyphae in a fluid medium obtained from below the mycelium at the stage of its highest rate of penicillin production and freed from impurities.' It was said to contain antibacterial agents which were removed during the purification. That such useful products might be lost during the purification step was later to be further emphasized when only partially purified extracts were found to have a wider therapeutic spectrum than the purified product. Judging from the following quote, Vivicillin proved reasonably successful: 'No extravagant claims or comparisons are made, for like penicillin, it is not a cure-all. However, very promising recoveries following its local and general use have taken place in medical and surgical patients, either when used alone where other known modern remedies have been used and have failed, and in combination with other modern remedies, the action of which it appears to accelerate.'

Vivicillin was produced on a commercial scale by the Watford Chemical Company; later, it was to undergo extensive clinical trials and was ultimately to be considered of little true value. Florey was clearly of the opinion that Vivicillin and its relative Penatin were of no value. In a reply to a letter from a Brazilian doctor sent as late as June 1951, he wrote:

> You do not state where this stuff has been made, but it may be similar to material made in this country and sold under the name Vivicillin and Penatin. As far as I know these products are worthless. It has never been demonstrated that they have any real antibacterial action. I suspect that the product that you have sent in your ampoules is of doubtful value; as you remark, the scientific basis for the use of such a product is not strong. If I were ill I would prefer to have some genuine penicillin.

Without doubt the most interesting and surprising development in the use of crude penicillin came in October 1943, when two Professors of Pathology at Queensland University, Australia, saved the life of a woman dying from septicaemia by administering injections of crude penicillin. The doctors, Duhigg and Grey, gave the woman a massive dose of 300 millilitres (nearly half a pint) of crude penicillin, and at the end of the treatment, some 5 litres of the crude material had been passed into the blood stream of this 42-year old Brisbane woman!

Finally, it seems that an unknown member of Florey's team became involved in the production and use of penicillin as early as 1940. In that year, an article by Dr H. S. Frazer in the *British Medical Journal* reports that Florey invited a Barbadian to Oxford in 1939. The man returned to Barbados in 1940, where he apparently grew *P. notatum* in Gordon's gin bottles and began to treat patients with crude penicillin!

There is no doubt that crude penicillin could have alleviated much suffering and saved lives, providing a useful stop gap until the infinitely more effective purified product became more widely available. There is, however, a cautionary rider to this optimistic view, since as early as 1942, a team of doctors at the Johns Hopkins Hospital in Baltimore, led by John E. Bordley, became aware of the fact that while crude penicillin was effective in killing staphylococci, streptococci and pneumococci, certain strains of all of these organisms showed resistance, and some could even grow in broth containing relatively high concentrations of the crude product. As we shall see in a later chapter, bacterial resistance to purified penicillin would develop rapidly following its widespread use in medicine. It is possible, therefore, that had crude penicillin continued to be used, perhaps on a larger scale, it would have led to an increase in the spread of bacteria. This is because the amount of active ingredient in the crude material would have been insufficient to kill all bacteria, and some would have developed resistance, perhaps to the point where they would have become unaffected by purified penicillin.

5

Penicillin: Personalities
and Conflicts

During 1944, rumours began to circulate that the Nobel Prize for physiology or medicine would be awarded that year for the discovery of penicillin. It was initially assumed that Fleming alone would be offered the Prize and that Florey and Chain would be ignored. In the end justice prevailed and all three shared the Prize, 'for the discovery of penicillin and its curative effects on various diseases.'

Few developments in science have been so widely written about as the discovery of penicillin, and despite the fact that Fleming's discovery was made over 50 years ago, interest in the history of penicillin shows no signs of waning. A major biography of Fleming has recently appeared, while there are at least four English-language biographies of Florey and a recent one has also been devoted to Chain. Interest in penicillin obviously reflects its dramatic impact on medicine, but also something more. The story is amazingly complex and contains a variety of interesting characters, from the taciturn Fleming to the more volatile Chain, while the enigmatic figure of Howard Florey provides that essential quality of intrigue.

In popular mythology, the credit for the discovery and development of penicillin is given solely to Fleming, while little if any credit is given to the Oxford group. Recently, however, there has been a determined attempt to try and correct this imbalance, to the point where Fleming's role in the discovery is now being played down. This 'counter-revolution' is aimed at destroying what has come to be known as the 'Fleming Myth'.

There is no doubt that Fleming has received too much of the credit for penicillin, but to a large extent the responsibility for this lay with Florey. It was Florey who made the decision to avoid the limelight and shun any publicity for the role of the Oxford group in the development of penicillin. In the early years of the last war, the general public was in desperate need of some good news and the discovery of penicillin provided a welcome alternative to the general gloom and despondency. It was not surprising that the discoverers of this miraculous wonder drug should be the target of idolatry. Florey chose to avoid this, while Fleming, approaching the end of his career, was more than happy to enjoy the adulation and new-found trappings of success.

Although Fleming was not directly involved in the development of his own myth, he never went out of his way to correct some of its wilder manifestations. Perhaps he felt that it was the responsibility of the Oxford Professor to fight his own corner. The following report, from *The Times*, 2 October 1947, on a speech made by Fleming when he opened the Pharmaceutical College in 1947, shows that he did not take the 'myth' at all seriously:

> There had been many stories in the newspapers about the origin of penicillin. There was one about the gentle breeze wafting a mould spore onto a plate. There was another where a bomb dropped and blew it in. This one was about ten years ahead of its time. The next one said that it was through his absent mindedness, because he took sandwiches every day to the hospital and apparently one day forgot to eat his lunch. A fortnight afterwards, he ate the sandwich which had gone mouldy. At that time, again according to the story, he was suffering from boils, which were miraculously cured!

Fleming has often been described as a genius. While I don't believe that this is the case, he was nevertheless a representative of a very special type of scientist, of which one sees few examples today. Fleming was a great observer, who took an almost childlike delight in the study of microorganisms. This is not to say that he was some kind of dilettante who spent his time merely *playing* with bacteria. Although he rarely put forward a hypothesis and then checked it by experimentation, Fleming was always quick to see, and then act upon, what was apparently obvious, but was missed by others. Nowadays scientists often downgrade such observational skills, and as a result Fleming is often described as merely an *observer*, as if this represented some low level of scientific endeavour.

Few scientific works have been subjected to such close scrutiny as has Fleming's first paper on penicillin. In style and scientific content the paper owes much to a similar one published in 1915 by Leonard Colebrook. It has come in for a considerable amount of criticism, a lot of it surprisingly uninformed. However, there is little doubt that this paper was one of the best and most thorough contributions to appear up to 1929 on the subject of microbial antagonism. While the paper contains a number of errors and omissions it is nevertheless quite sound, as is evidenced by the ease with which Chain was able to repeat Fleming's findings.

Fleming has been criticized on a number of counts in relation to this paper. Firstly it is said that the few references given at the end demonstrate that he was unaware of the vast literature which was by then available on the subject of microbial antagonism. However, Fleming could hardly have been unaware of this literature. He probably regarded the penicillin phenomenon as being distinct from the usual examples of microbial antagonism, because of the all-important occurrence of bacterial lysis, rather than merely inhibition. There is a more prosaic reason why Fleming kept to a minimum the number of references he gave to early work on microbial antagonism. He was simply following the editors' instructions, which demanded that authors limit historical references to a minimum. These instructions also require that authors avoid excessive speculation, a fact which perhaps explains why Fleming failed to discuss at length his ideas on how penicillin might be used in medicine. The editorial instructions are to be found on the inside of the front cover of the *British Journal Of Experimental Pathology*, which is invariably removed before being bound into library copies. As a result Fleming's critics have missed the obvious reasons for the omissions in his paper, and have consequently drawn many wrong conclusions concerning his motives.

A criticism which is frequently levelled against Fleming is that he failed to fully appreciate penicillin's therapeutic potential, particularly in relation to the possibility that it might prove curative when injected into the bloodstream. However, in the period immediately following the penicillin discovery, Fleming had not been exposed to the dramatic change in the climate of medical opinion brought about by the introduction of the sulphonamides. As far as Fleming and his contemporaries were concerned, the idea of injecting an antiseptic into the bloodstream was a non-starter. To criticize Fleming for this attitude is like criticizing the Wright brothers for not having envisaged space flight!

As we have seen, Fleming did attempt to use penicillin to cure infections, and the best reply that can be given to his critics is to ask: if the therapeutic potential of penicillin was so obvious, why did Fleming's contemporaries, including Florey and Hare, not queue up to have a go at purifying it and then use it to cure patients? The medical world was, after all, desperate for a curative like penicillin and it is inconceivable that had the idea of using it in this way been obvious it would have lain unnoticed for so long.

A comment by Ronald Hare, in relation to his work with Colebrook on penicillin, gives us an insight as to why penicillin was neglected in this way:

> Penicillin was of course discussed. It could not very well be ignored. But it was at about this time that the paper by Clutterbuck and co-workers appeared. The mere fact that expert chemists, in so well an appointed laboratory as the School of Hygiene, had stopped studying penicillin because it appeared to disappear into thin air when an ether solution was allowed to evaporate, sounded its death knell as far as we were concerned. We had neither the time nor the staff to pursue what seemed no more than a will o' the wisp, or as some put it about that time, one of Flem's foolish fantasies.

Fleming expressed almost exactly the same sentiments, but still his critics fail to grasp the historical context of his work, and unfairly castigate him for not having done more to purify penicillin and apply it in medicine.

While the 'Fleming Myth' has been extensively commented upon, less has been said about what we might refer to as the 'Oxford Myth'. This takes the following form: some time in 1938, Chain studied the literature on microbial antagonism, with a view to pursuing some purely academic work on microbial antagonism, when, out of the blue, he came upon penicillin. Then Florey with amazing insight suggested that Chain concentrate on this substance. Again there was no thought of applying this work to a medical use for penicillin. The Oxford team then purified penicillin and gave it to the world as the first effective antibiotic. At this point Fleming reappeared and stole the glory for penicillin.

Like the 'Fleming Myth', the Oxford variety is full of truth and falsehood, but unlike the former this myth has largely gone unchallenged. To begin with, we have already seen that Florey was well aware of penicillin from the time of its discovery, and he knew from his conversations with Paine that it could be used to cure infections. Yet he did nothing to promote its use in medicine. In fact, in retrospect, we can see that Florey maintained an interest in penicillin from the moment Fleming reported its discovery in 1929. Bickel, in his biography of Florey, *Rise Up To Life*, states that in 1929 Florey even suggested to the Oxford bacteriologist Dr E. G. D. Murray that he might try to purify penicillin, but Murray declined because he believed that his knowledge of biochemistry was not up to the task. It was as if fate had determined that he was to play a major role in the development of penicillin. Bickel summarizes this view in the following words: 'From 1929 onwards, when Fleming published his paper on the *Penicillium* mould, Florey had been on the path of penicillin by way of lysozyme, and nothing would have diverted him from that course.'

In addition, the relationship between Florey and Chain appears to have often been far from ideal, and Chain never seems to have accepted the view that the purification of penicillin was a team effort. The rift between Florey and Chain appears to have been opened when Florey took Heatley, rather than Chain, to the US to seek the support of the American pharmaceutical industry. Chain took this as a direct personal insult, although, in truth, Heatley, with his greater knowledge of the practicalities of penicillin production, was by far the better choice. The following words of Chain show how deeply slighted he felt that he was not chosen to travel to the US with Florey:

> He did not tell me of any action he took to arrange a journey to the U.S.A. and the first time I heard that he was going, accompanied by Heatley, was when I entered his office one day (I think in the spring) of 1941 for a routine talk and found his suitcases standing on the floor packed for the journey. When I asked him where he was going he told me that Heatley and he were leaving for the U.S.A. in half an hour. No other word of explanation came from him. I left the room silently but shattered by the experience of this underhand trick and act of bad faith, the worst so far in my experience of Florey. It spoiled my initially good relations with this man forever.'

Chain, it seems, also felt hard done by, as if Florey had stolen some of the credit that was due to him. However, Chain himself was also to be surrounded by his own mythology. In particular, it is usually assumed that it was his brilliant abilities as a biochemist which brought about the rapid purification of penicillin at Oxford. In fact, as we have already seen, it was Heatley who made the important suggestion that penicillin be transferred back from solvent into water or buffer. Chain pooh-poohed this suggestion, partly because he was still labouring under the idea that penicillin was an enzyme.

There seems little doubt that Florey was slow to appreciate the importance of penicillin, and he only really appears to have become totally committed to the research programme following the results of the first mouse-protection tests. Having recognized penicillin's potential, however, he worked tirelessly to get it into mass production. Florey without doubt provided the vital energy and drive behind the development of penicillin as an effective antibiotic.

My comments on what I have described as the 'Oxford Myth' are in no way intended to denigrate the magnificent work done by Florey and his associates. I have included them to show how easy it is, given the benefit of hindsight, to single out any one of the penicillin pioneers for criticism. To date most of this unwarranted criticism has been directed towards Fleming. But his contribution was obviously fundamental. After all, it was he who discovered penicillin and wrote the paper which enabled Chain to get a head start with its purification. Penicillin would no doubt eventually have been discovered without Fleming, although it is unlikely that Florey and Chain would have been involved, or that penicillin would have been available in time to contribute to the Allied victory in the Second World War.

The Relationship between Fleming and Florey

Whatever ill-feelings were later to develop between Fleming and Florey, their initial relationship was good to the point of being friendly. This is clearly shown in correspondence between the two held in the Florey Archive. We have seen that Fleming visited Florey in Oxford on 2 September 1940, and that they began to correspond with one another about penicillin. Fleming forwarded a number of variants of his penicillin-producing mould in the hope that they would prove superior to the original, while Florey responded by giving Fleming a sample of the Oxford penicillin. An exchange of friendly letters about the Lambert case then occurred, culminating in a letter from Fleming stating that: 'We are all here very grateful to you for your kindness in letting us have penicillin which in this case undoubtedly saved the Man's life.'

Up until the summer of 1942, then, there seems to have existed a friendly, professional relationship between the two men, but this state of affairs was not to last much longer. On 29 August, 1942, Florey wrote to Fleming saying: 'You will have noticed in the *Times* some very undesirable press publicity. I have done my best to stop this sort of thing but I was not asked about this particular case.' Florey then lists the contribution which the Oxford team made to the development of penicillin, obviously pointing out the error in assigning the credit for its development as a useable drug to Fleming. On the 2 September Fleming replies, going onto the defensive: 'I was glad to see Robinson's letter in the *Times* this morning. Although my luck started you off on the penicillin hunt, it is you who have made it a practical proposition and so it is good that you should get the credit.' It is a pity that these or similar words were not widely publicized as they would have gone a long way to defuse the acrimony which was later to develop. Up to this point, then, it is clear that Fleming was keen to share the credit for penicillin with Florey. He ends his letter by bemoaning the press reporters who continually pestered him and misrepresented his statements:

> You cannot deplore the personal element which has crept into penicillin more than I do and for the moment I am the sufferer. I was out in the Sector all day last Friday and when I got back in the late afternoon Wright told me he had been rung up by some weekly review that he had never heard of. On Saturday morning when I arrived in the lab. I found the *News Chronicle* people planted on my bench. I hated it and I have been suffering since. The photograph looks like I was really suffering – where it came from I have no idea but it is not one I myself would have chosen. The *Illustrated London News* rang up last week and said that they were publishing an article on penicillin. I was told that it had been carefully prepared from our published articles and that there was none of the press ballyhoo ... I do hope that the people who matter (the others do not count) do not think we are in opposition. I will certainly do what I can to dispel the idea if it exists. As you say, our contributions are perfectly clear cut and complementary and no-one can accuse me of ever having said that my work was not acknowledged ...

On the evidence of this letter there was clearly no sign that Fleming was out to deny Florey his share of the penicillin glory. Nevertheless, antagonism, of the human kind, continued to develop between the two penicillin pioneers. For example, as early as 1942, Florey wrote to Sir Henry Dale, then the President of the Royal Society, that: 'I have now quite good evidence, from the director-general of the BBC in fact, and also from some people at St Mary's, that Fleming is doing his best to see the whole subject is presented as having been foreseen and worked out by Fleming and that we in this department just did a few final flourishes.' Chain, on the other hand, took a more practical stance on the question of Fleming's apparent attempts to steal the penicillin limelight: 'the British hospitals,' he wrote, 'were struggling for their pennies remember. Then here, suddenly, was a pot of gold for St Mary's. It was an opportunity to be grasped – and if I had been the manager of the hospital, I might have done the same.' However, Chain too could be annoyed by the public manifestations of the Fleming myth. While visiting the States in 1945, he wrote to Florey:

> The Oxford work is of course never mentioned by him [Fleming]. It will take a great deal of very considerable effort to get things into their proper perspectives, and I will do what I can though I am under no illusions about the difficulties and delicacy inherent in the present situation. I came here fully prepared to find the usual distortions of the history of the penicillin discovery, but I must confess that I was staggered to see how far these distortions have gone through the systematic and carefully planned efforts of Fleming.

An equally revealing series of correspondence, this time between Florey and his old friend John Fulton, is also preserved in the Florey Archive. This material is particularly useful since it provides an alternative view on why the relationship between Fleming and Florey became so strained. Fulton wrote to Florey on 6 January 1944 saying:

> My only concern is that some well meaning people seem to think that Fleming, to whom you have been so very generous deserves the chief credit. Actually Fleming observed what my house officers have observed for the last 20 years, namely that when a culture of pathogens become contaminated with mould the growth of the pathogenic colonies is inhibited. Fleming did make a small technical application of the observation, but the wider implications he utterly failed to see.

Fulton was obviously showing his ignorance of the special nature of the penicillin phenomenon when he wrote these words, and was also clearly not giving Fleming his due.

In another letter written later that year, Fulton no longer refers to Fleming by name, preferring the somewhat derisory notation 'F'. There is clear evidence in this letter that Fulton, and perhaps Florey, is now definitely beginning to view Fleming as one of the enemy. In the letter, Fulton bemoans the fact that 'there has been an ever mounting emphasis in the local press on the importance of 'F's' contribution', and 'the adroit Scot has talked our drug house people out of eighty thousand dollars for St Mary's.'

Doubtless Fulton was responding to Florey's mounting feeling that his role in the penicillin story was being increasingly ignored. Fulton's response was that of a good friend, but in trying to argue that Fleming should not share in the Nobel Prize his actions went beyond the bounds of one friend helping another. When approached by the Swedish legation in New York, Fulton suggested the first choice for the prize should be Florey alone, or if this was not acceptable, then Florey and Chain, while his last preference was the Oxford two plus Fleming. Fulton incorrectly stated that this order of preference 'represented the considered opinion of a large group in this country [that is the US], including the Division of Medical Sciences of the National Research Council and Officers of the American Medical Association'.

Fortunately, the Nobel Prize Committee realized that these views were not, in fact, typical of US medical opinion, and Fulton's last option, which no one could argue was unfair, was the one selected. However, Fulton seems to have been contented by the fact that his friend was awarded the Prize, since he was to send a telegram including the words 'all's well that ends well'.

Many of the problems which arose concerning the allocation of credit for the discovery might have been avoided had the Oxford team decided to call the purified product by a different name. Fleming used the term penicillin to refer to the antibacterial filtrates of a certain mould. Some have argued that Florey would have been justified in using an alternative name for the therapeutic derivative from these filtrates. An attempt was in fact made to introduce the term 'therapeutic penicillin' to the Oxford product but, presumably because it was unwieldy, the term never caught on. As a result, 'penicillin' continued to mean both the crude filtrates and the highly purified product, and an opportunity was missed to help differentiate between Fleming's discovery and the later Oxford work.

The personal antagonism which had developed between Fleming and Florey over recognition for the penicillin discovery can be appreciated from the following letter which was sent by Florey in November 1945 to an American, Miss Flora Kaplin. Miss Kaplin, it seems, was contemplating writing a book on the penicillin story and wrote to Florey for his advice. The reply was as follows:

> I shall be very glad if, in writing your book, you would make it absolutely clear that there was no connection between Sir Alexander Fleming and Dr Chain and myself. Sir Alexander Fleming works at St Mary's Hospital, London; Dr Chain and I work at the Sir William Dunn School of Pathology at Oxford. Dr Chain and I were not co-workers with Sir Alexander Fleming in any sense of the word and it is a gross misrepresentation, which seems to have acquired wide

currency, to say that we were. Sir Alexander Fleming's work on penicillin ceased in 1932 until he took it up again after the main body of the work had been done in Oxford. I should be indebted if you were to leave your readers under no illusion on this point.

The problems which arose between Fleming and Florey were to a large extent the product of Florey's decision to stay aloof from the publicity for penicillin, a decision, incidentally, which Chain never appreciated since it meant that he too was denied a full share of the 'spoils'. Such problems could have been avoided had Florey and Fleming published a joint statement of their respective roles in the development of penicillin, or perhaps if they had appeared on a platform together. Unfortunately, except at the Nobel Prize Ceremony, this never happened. Instead Fleming provided the focus for public idolatry, and for that he has been criticized by some ever since.

Perhaps Chain should have the last word on the subject of the penicillin discovery. It is true to say that, for some years, Chain did not regard Fleming very highly, and he was not particularly impressed by the role that the Scottish bacteriologist had played in the discovery of penicillin. In later life, however, he came to a more balanced view of Fleming's discovery. In 1979, he ended an article which he wrote concerning Fleming's contribution with the following words: 'We ourselves at Oxford, in the discovery of the curative properties of penicillin, had plenty of luck. Therefore it is petty and irrelevant to try to detract from the importance of Fleming's discovery by ascribing it entirely to good luck, and there is no doubt that this discovery, which has changed the history of medicine, has justly earned him a position of immortality.'

6

Penicillin after the War

PENICILLIN: THE DREAM BEGINS TO FADE

In 1947, an American woman was given an injection of penicillin, apparently without any ill effects. In August of the following year she was given a second dose of the antibiotic, after which she complained of a strange taste in her mouth, which was later accompanied by a swelling in her throat. Then, while leaning over the kitchen table, she suddenly collapsed and died. This was the first fatality ascribed to penicillin, but unfortunately it was not to prove the last.

It seems that even despite its remarkably low toxicity some people develop an allergy to penicillin, and in some cases this allergic response can cause death. The first examples of these deaths were to be reported in the popular US magazine, the *Coronet*, during 1949. The article appeared under the title, 'The Truth About Wonder Drugs'. It went a long way towards destroying the myth that penicillin was infallible, pointing out that some people could develop a fatal allergy to penicillin even if they had not been previously exposed to the drug.

In the four years from 1953, 81 people died from penicillin-associated allergy in the US alone, figures which need, of course, to be set against the many millions of people who received the antibiotic, and also against the large number of lives it saved. Deaths in England and Wales due to penicillin-hypersensitivity, for example, occurred at a rate of only 1 per 10 million of the population! This statistic can be put into perspective by individual tragedies, as can be seen from the following cases. In 1957, an Oxford farmer was admitted into the Radcliffe Infirmary, the home of the first penicillin triumphs. He was given an injection of penicillin, to which he was known to be sensitive, and died. His widow received £12,500 in damages for what was only 1 of the 20 penicillin-related deaths which then occurred annually in the UK alone. In the second example, a 24-year old man died after receiving a dose of penicillin 500 times greater than that recommended to treat the meningitis from which he was suffering.

Penicillin-hypersensitivity was eventually found to be linked to the use of unnecessarily high dose rates, so a reduction in the amount prescribed, and the recognition of those at risk, soon reduced the small number of cases of penicillin fatalities. Nevertheless, comments in the *Coronet* such as 'the wonder drug becomes blunder drug', and 'penicillin turns killer', reflected the growing realization that penicillin was not to be the first infallible troublefree drug in the history of medicine.

As early as 1942, another problem with penicillin began to be recognized for the first time. In that year, the first penicillin-resistant strains of *Staphylococcus aureus* were isolated. These strains were shown by Abraham and Chain to be capable of producing the enzyme 'penicillinase' which destroyed penicillin, thereby making the bacteria resistant. These resistant strains then spread to other patients and many doctors and nurses themselves became carriers. Such spread of penicillin-resistant bacteria took place with amazing speed. Only 12 per cent of the staphylococci isolated from patients in the Hammersmith Hospital in London during 1946 were found to be resistant to penicillin, a figure which rose to 38 and 59 per cent respectively in each of the following years.

The rapid development of this penicillin resistance obviously had an impact on diseases, some of which had been on the point of being completely controllable using penicillin. For example, penicillin treatment reduced fatalities caused by staphylococcal infections to 28 per cent by 1945, but in the years from 1951–3, this figure had increased to 54 per cent, to reach an amazing 80 per cent by the years from 1953 to 1955!

Today, however, by careful attention to aseptic technique and with the help of new antistaphylococcal antibiotics and penicillinase inhibitors, doctors have reached an uneasy equilibrium, in which the spread of antibiotic-resistant bacteria is kept to a minimum. In the penultimate chapter, however, we will see that bacterial resistance to penicillin and the other antibiotics continues to be a major problem in our hospitals.

'OFF THE SHELF' PENICILLINS

It is perhaps not surprising that many of the British and US pharmaceutical companies were at first reluctant to commit themselves to penicillin production by fermentation. The pharmaceutical industry could reflect that as late as 1938 the Lederle Division of the American Cyanamid Company had lost millions of dollars when a new plant for the production of pneumonia vaccines was made obsolete by the appearance of sulphapyridine. The risks involved in producing penicillin by the relatively novel technology of fermentation were obvious, especially since it was assumed that penicillin would very soon be chemically synthesized on an industrial scale. Merck, in particular, took this view and when large-scale penicillin synthesis failed to materialize, they lost out in a major way to their competitors who had backed fermentation production.

Before penicillin could be synthesized it was necessary first to crystallize it and then to determine its chemical structure. When this crystallization was eventually achieved, it was found that penicillin, rather than being a single entity, could exist in a number of forms. The Oxford material was found to be distinct from the US product, and was given the name penicillin I, later to be changed to penicillin F. The US penicillin was at first referred to as penicillin G, but was later to become better known as benzyl penicillin.

Then, in 1945, Dorothy Hodgkin, working at Oxford, made the all-important discovery that penicillin possessed a β lactam ring. Once the structure of penicillin was established, it was hoped that synthesis would not be far away. One of the leading Merck scientists involved in the search for this synthesis was John Sheenan, who, after leaving Merck, continued this work when he became Professor of Chemistry at the Massachusetts Institute of Technology. In 1957, Sheenan synthesized penicillin V, but could only produce trace quantities. This synthesis led to the preparation of 6-aminopenicillanic acid, again only in small quantities, but it proved to be the key to the production of penicillins containing new side chains. Then, in 1958, Batchelor and co-workers at Beecham, helped by suggestions from Chain, prepared 4-aminopenicillin G from which it was confidently expected that new penicillins would be produced. Beecham then took out a patent on the large-scale production of 6-aminopenicillanic acid, and entered into licensing agreements with Bristol Laboratories, the company who had funded Sheenan's work. At first all went well, until the inevitable squabbles arose over patent rights.

The synthesis of these new penicillins allowed the inadequacies of penicillin G to be overcome. In 1948 Lilly introduced penicillin V which, unlike benzyl penicillin, was not destroyed in the stomach, and so could be taken by mouth. This then led to the introduction of the first effective oral penicillin, V-Cil-K.

Semi-synthetic penicillins like methicillin, a compound resistant to β

lactamase, then followed. In 1961, Beecham introduced an orally active variant of methicillin called oxacillin, to be followed by cloxacillin, flucloxacillin and dichloroxacillin – all antibiotics which are now reserved for the fight against penicillin-resistant staphylococci.

Beecham then went on to produce the first broad-spectrum penicillin, ampicillin. Unfortunately, this penicillin was susceptible to β lactamase and was poorly absorbed by the gut. This led to some patients suffering acute diarrhoea, because the unabsorbed ampicillin interfered with the ecological interrelationships of the normal gut microflora. The closely related amoxycillin, which had better adsorption characteristics was introduced in 1964, to be followed by pivampicillin. In that same year, carbencillin and ticacillin, antibiotics with marked activity against *Pseudomonas aeuruginosa*, were introduced. These proved particularly effective for use in burns patients suffering from infections caused by this bacterium. As a result of these synthetic penicillins doctors can now keep one step ahead in the fight against infection. Penicillin now comes as a whole range of antibiotics with individual properties, which enable the physician to target their use to a specific medical problem.

THE IMPACT OF PENICILLIN ON MEDICINE

Penicillin's impact on medicine can by gauged by the fact that, in 1979, some 15,000 tons of fermented bulk product were produced, having a minimum market value of 240 million dollars. Most of these fermentation products were then converted into semi-synthetic penicillins with a market value of a staggering 1,250 million dollars! Just 50 years after the appearance of Fleming's first penicillin paper, there was sufficient penicillin produced to give a 5 gramme dose to every man, woman and child on the planet!

Penicillin had a dramatic effect on infection and mortality resulting from bacterial infections, such as staphylococcal and puerperal sepsis, pneumococcal pneumonia, otitis media and bacterial meningitis. It also had a big impact on minor diseases, such as impetigo, which as a result is rarely seen nowadays (although the incidence of this infection is beginning to increase in some parts of the world due to the appearance of resistant bacterial strains). Just as importantly, the advent of penicillin allowed for major advances to be made in surgery, allowing for organ transplantation, cardiac surgery and the efficient management of severe burns.

Today penicillin is no longer a single product but is a range of compounds having differing properties and uses. Modern penicillins can be broadly divided into benzyl penicillin, penicillinase-stable penicillins, broad-spectrum and anti-pseudomonal penicillins. Benzyl penicillins are still the antibiotic of choice for the treatment of puerperal fever, pyogenic meningitis, syphilis, gas gangrene, gonorrhea and pneumonia. These penicillins are, however, poorly absorbed by the stomach, and with the exception of penicillin V cannot be given by mouth. Three penicillinase-stable penicillins are widely used in the UK, namely methicillin, cloxacillin and flucloxacillin. Broad-spectrum penicillins are effective against Gram-negative bacteria such as *E. coli*, *Shigella* and *Salmonella* . Unfortunately this class of compounds is often abused as a panacea for all ills.

The many different types of penicillins remain amongst the safest drugs a doctor can prescribe, and all, including the original benzyl penicillin, remain extremely valuable antibiotics. The first miracle of the penicillin story is the antibiotic itself which, with its undreamt of healing powers, changed the course of medicine. The second miracle is the speed at which penicillin was transformed from a laboratory oddity to an inexpensive mass-produced antibiotic. In 1942, there was barely enough penicillin to treat 100 patients, yet, by 1958, 400 tons of crystalline penicillin were produced in the US alone, a state of affairs which the penicillin pioneers could hardly have imagined in their wildest dreams!

7

The Road to Antibiotics

Archaeologists studying the remains of a tribe who lived in Sudanese Nubia around 350 AD made a surprising discovery. During investigations of the remains of these people they found evidence for traces of tetracycline. This antibiotic was thought to have first been discovered in the mid-1940s, yet here were traces of it in the bones of an ancient people. It seems that these people must have been ingesting small amounts of tetracycline over a long period, and the most likely explanation is that tetracycline-producing *Streptomyces* contaminated the food grains which they stored in mud-lined bins, and from there entered their daily bread. There remains the possibility, however, that certain witches or elders knew of the curative effects of these contaminated grains and purposely provided the conditions which would promote the growth of a specific bacterium or mould. This may explain why this group appear to have suffered a lower incidence of infectious disease than other primitive peoples living around the same time.

Ample evidence exists to suggest that mould therapy was used from antiquity to relatively modern times to treat wounds and infections. The Chinese of 3,000 years ago, for example, are thought to have applied mouldy soya beans to skin infections, while the Egyptian Papyrus Hearst, which is assigned to the eighteenth dynasty (around 1500 BC), details similar mould cures in prescriptions numbered 189–92. Reference to mould cures is also given in the Jewish Talmud, and in the folk medicine of Europe and the Americas. An English herbal of 1760, for example, refers to the use of mouldy bread to treat infected wounds, while John Parkinson, apothecary of London and the King's herbalist, advised a similar treatment in 1640. In many Cornish and Devonshire farmhouses a loaf of bread, called the 'Good Friday Bun', was, in earlier ages, allowed to go mouldy and then used throughout the rest of the year as a curative.

A recent reference to this treatment was given in a letter to the *Sunday Express* (19 March 1989) by a Reverend J. Aelwyn Roberts in the following words:

> And yet there is nothing new under the sun. Penicillin [sic] was used in parts of Yorkshire up to the end of the last century. Here it was custom on Good Friday or on Maundy Thursday to bake a few more hot cross buns than the family could reasonably eat. These were put away in a suitable container and allowed to grow mouldy. Some time near Pentecost the mould would be scraped off the buns and put into a jar and for the rest of the year the hot cross bun ointment would be used as a cure all for all cuts and abrasions.

Similar references to mould cures can also be found in the folklore of the Americas, the Far East and Africa. For example, in 1911, a doctor in North Carolina, John Bricknell, described how an Indian witch doctor took the rotten grains of maize or Indian corn, 'well dried and beaten to powder', and used it to cure an ulcer on a white man's leg. This is an interesting reference because it may be explained by the ability of some penicillia to produce an antibacterial agent called penicillic acid when growing on maize. In a similar vein, Lyall Watson, in his book *Supernature* refers to a South African tribe, the Pedi, who apparently believed that infections could be cured by using a con- coction made from grain which had been chewed by a cross-eyed child and then hung from the branches of a certain tree which grew close to water, when the grains became covered with a mould. Such moulds may then have produced an antibacterial metabolite, although one wonders whether it was necessary to employ the services of a cross- eyed child to achieve this effect!

Many relatively recent uses of mould therapy have been cited by people who were children in the pre-antibiotic era. Here is one such account which was recently sent to me by a Dr McMally from Cork in Ireland:

> Many years ago an old aunt (who was some 82 years old) who appeared to be quite learned in cures read one day in a magazine of Professor Fleming's discovery of penicillin, which was described as resulting from research on mould. My aunt said in her inimitable way, '*I had that cure before he*

did'. I know that one of her cures was to collect ten or twelve oranges and place them somewhere where they would get mouldy as soon as possible. She would then carefully remove the greenest mould and make it into some kind of infusion and use it on abscesses, whitlows, boils or other forms of pustule. She would then administer it orally, all apparently with complete success.

In a similar vein, a Mrs L. Collingwood of Hull provided me with this account:

> My grandfather, when I was young and used to stay with them (mid to late 1920s) and if we had nasty sore knees, grit and scabs from falling down, he used to get his penknife and cut and scrape the ham or bacon side hung from the ceiling (to be cured), salted and green with mould and put the fat on a piece of clean linen and Grandma used to wrap our knees up and it always cleansed and healed our wounds.

One final example will suffice to demonstrate how extensive were experiences of the pre-antibiotic use of the curative properties of moulds. This one was related by A. W. Somerville of Bournemouth and published as a letter in the *Sunday Telegraph* on 26 August 1979:

> It must have been in the early years of this century, when I, as a little boy, developed poisoned legs. The front of each leg seemed to be a mass of yellow blisters from knee to ankle. My parents tried every cure as did our family doctor without success, and in desperation my mother asked nurse Exelby, who lived next door, if she could help. Here is her prescription:
>
> 1. Toast a pure linen handkerchief before the fire until lightly browned.
> 2. Take the mould from off the top of raspberry jam and spread it evenly over the handkerchief and apply to each leg.
> 3. Bandage each leg securely and put the boy to bed, so that the dressing will not be moved.
>
> When the dressings were removed – I should think with more hope than expectation – I can remember a strange look on my parents' faces and then a hesitant laugh and few tears from my mother. The wounds appeared almost clear of

infection. Whether a second dressing was necessary I cannot say, but certainly there were no more than two.

A response to this letter by W. H. Cousins of Essex confirms the widespread use of such therapy when he states: 'I must point out to A. W. Somerville, who wrote of the curative properties of raspberry jam mould, that mouldy bread as a dressing for sores was known for generations before Sir Alexander Fleming independently discovered the curative properties of the mould.'

Bakers' and brewers' yeast have also been used since antiquity to treat surface infections, and as early as 1909, Fernbach noted that yeasts produced substances toxic to other yeasts, filamentous fungi and bacteria. The likely scientific rationale behind the folk use of yeast was confirmed in 1941 by Cook and co-workers who showed that alcoholic extracts of bakers' yeast inhibited *E. coli*, *Staphylococcus aureus* and fungi like *Aspergillus niger* and *Penicillium glaucum*. Complete killing of none of these organisms was obtained, but growth rates were greatly depressed by 2 per cent or more.

Most medical historians have tended to dismiss these claims for the curative properties of moulds as merely old wives' tales; however, the fact that such practices took place on all continents and in all ages suggests that they must to some extent have been successful. Where claims for the effectiveness of these folk-cures have been accepted it has generally been assumed that the agent involved must have been penicillin. However, while this may have been the case, a more likely contender is a compound called patulin. Patulin, about which we will hear more later, is an antibacterial agent which is produced by a variety of moulds found growing on various foodstuffs. It is too toxic to be used in medicine but, as it is a very common product of mould growth, it probably accounts for the apparent effectiveness of mould therapies.

Many of the products of mould growth on grains are mycotoxins and when ingested over long periods may cause liver damage or even perhaps cancer. Our forebears may, therefore, have been extremely careful when using this approach to therapy. If they did not know the conditions which favoured the growth of non-toxic moulds, then the long-term ingestion of mycotoxins must have helped cause many premature deaths.

As late as 1925, an editorial in the *Lancet* made the following perceptive reference to the use of fungi in medicine: 'Medicinal properties attributed by tradition to certain fungi may possibly represent an untapped source of therapeutic virtue.' Whatever the merits, or otherwise, of these ancient cures, one thing is for certain: the discovery of penicillin in no way depended on what had gone before. Indeed, had

Fleming or anyone else admitted basing the discovery of an antibiotic on this folk medicine they would have exposed themselves to instant ridicule. Nevertheless, there had been, prior to Fleming's discovery, a long history of the scientific study of microbial antagonism and, as we have seen, attempts were even made to use this knowledge of the ability of one group of organisms to treat infections.

JAMES TWOMEY'S NOVEL APPROACH TO MOULD THERAPY

At about the same time as Cecil Paine began working with crude penicillin, another Sheffield doctor, James Twomey, was employing the therapeutic use of moulds, in a way analogous to the mouldy jam therapy described above in A. W. Somerville's letter. An excellent and convincing description of his methods was recently related to me by a Sheffield woman, Mrs Brenda Ward. Twomey was a junior partner in a family practice based at a surgery in Attercliffe, then a thriving district located in Sheffield's industrial heartland. In April 1929, Twomey used a mould preparation to treat Mrs Ward, then 8 years old and called Brenda Whitnear.

Brenda had contracted a severe case of impetigo. Her face, a small area of her elbow and the inside of her knee were covered with the characteristic dry, yellow crusts. Before the appearance of the sulphonamides and penicillin, this highly contagious disease, caused by *Staphylococcus aureus*, was a very common disease of childhood, which, if left untreated, could eventually cause complications such as liver damage. However, since the usual treatment was to keep children out of school and outside, playing in the fresh air, many probably welcomed a mild dose of impetigo.

Brenda's condition continued to worsen throughout the summer of 1929, to the point where she developed a high fever punctuated by bouts of delirium. Her ninth birthday passed, but despite the conventional treatment prescribed by her family doctor, Dr Kelly, her condition showed no signs of improvement. Dr Twomey was then brought in to give his opinion on the case.

Twomey had graduated from the University of Ireland in 1922 and following a short period as a general practitioner in Kanturk, County Cork, he moved to Sheffield in 1928. Twomey examined Brenda and then recommended a treatment which he described as a last resort. He told her mother to buy some ordinary domestic starch, of the hot water variety, and make it into a thick paste of about the same consistency as

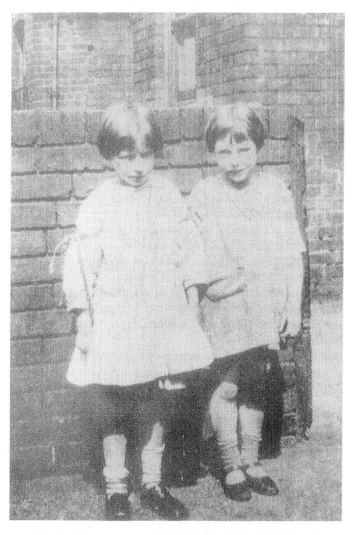

Plate 9 The young Brenda Whitnear (on the left), shortly
after being cured of impetigo by Dr James Twomey.
(Courtesy of Mrs B. Ward)

lemon curd. The starch was then to be left for three to four days in the
pantry at the head of the cellar, after which time he would return and
explain how the treatment was to proceed. On his return, Twomey
found, as he had expected, that the surface of the starch was covered in a
thick growth of green mould. He lifted the growth, examined it carefully

and then proclaimed that it was ready for use. Next, he told Brenda's mother to apply the starch paste to a face mask made from a pillow case. Brenda had been wearing such a mask whenever visitors came to see her, so as to hide the severity of her infection from them. The mould treatment continued until mid-August, by which time the impetigo had completely cleared, and Brenda was allowed to return to school in September.

The treatment was apparently inoffensive, despite 'itching mercilessly'. By chance, Mrs Ward has kept the doctor's receipt for the costs of her treatment, which came to 32s 13d for the period 9 April to 14 September 1929. Unfortunately the receipt gives no details of the treatment which was used. Mrs Ward can remember seeing the contaminated starch paste, and she describes it as being covered in what she calls 'rounds of mould growth, appearing pale yellow at first, then orange-brown and finally blue-green', in fact, a perfect lay-person's description of the growth of either a species of *Penicillium* or *Aspergillus*.

By a combination of deduction and a little detective work, the reasoning behind Twomey's treatment can be worked out. Firstly, why did he use a starch paste? This question is simple to answer: starch paste was widely used at that time to soften impetigo crusts prior to the application of an antiseptic. Secondly, from where did Twomey get the idea for his somewhat unorthodox treatment? He could of course have read Fleming's paper which appeared in June of the same year as he treated Brenda. However, he would have had little time to ask for a culture of Fleming's mould and do preliminary experiments on its effectiveness when inoculated into starch. In addition it is unlikely that Twomey, a general practitioner, would have read the specialist journal in which Fleming's paper appeared. A more likely possibility is that Twomey's methods were based on the folklore use of mould therapy. Since he was Irish by birth, it is not too fanciful to think that he had learned of this treatment in his native County Cork. The Irish connection would also make appropriate the choice of potato starch as a carrier for the mould. Finally, what was responsible for the apparent effectiveness of this treatment? It seems clear that the contaminating mould was able to produce some antibacterial metabolite while growing on the starch. To confirm this possibility, I repeated Twomey's experimental protocol as described by Mrs Ward and found that hot water starch does indeed tend to selectively isolate species of *Penicillium*. In addition, those that are isolated have the ability to inhibit *Staph. aureus*, the cause of impetigo. However, as we have already seen, this does not mean that Twomey's therapy necessarily relied upon the production of penicillin by a mould; more probably a metabolite like patulin was involved.

Twomey's mould therapy is quite distinct from the lineage of penicillin treatment begun by Fleming and independently continued by Paine. Most notably, it involved the use of a living mould, rather than a culture filtrate. As we have seen, however, live samples of *P. notatum* were later to be used in the 1940s to cure surface infections, a fact which points to the likely effectiveness of Twomey's treatment.

Sadly, Twomey was never to know of the miraculous effect which penicillin had on medicine. In May 1938 he left Hull, where he was then practising, to travel on business to London. Here, on Tuesday 17 May, he collapsed outside his hotel. He was rushed to hospital, but it was too late, and he died from what the *Hull Daily Mail* described as an 'affection of the throat'. Ironically, the hospital in which he died was St Mary's, and the infection which killed him would probably have been cured by penicillin.

Lysozyme: Fleming's First Major Discovery

Fleming spent the large part of his career researching into antiseptics, particularly with a view to using such compounds to defeat bacterial infections already established in the body. His studies on penicillin were in effect an extension of this work. Here was a natural antiseptic which he always maintained would eventually find a use in medicine. However, Fleming's experience as a doctor in the First World War had convinced him that antiseptics were not the answer to the problem of systemic bacterial infection since, when used on infected wounds, these agents interfered with the body's defence mechanism. During the war Fleming had written: 'Surrounded by all those infected wounds, by men who were suffering and dying without our being able to do anything to help them, I was consumed by a desire to discover, after all this struggling and waiting, something which would kill these microbes, something like Salvarsan.' These words adequately sum up Fleming's post-war career in scientific research. Much of this time, however, was to be wasted in an attempt to demonstrate the effectiveness of the concept called 'vaccine therapy', which was championed by Fleming's boss, Almroth Wright. Fleming was at first as convinced of the effectiveness of such treatment as was Wright, but as the years passed he began to lose faith in the value of the laborious daily round of tests. In the late 1930s, Fleming would turn to research on the sulphonamides, no doubt in the hope that the perfect antibacterial agent had at last arrived. It is somewhat ironic that for something like ten years he unknowingly had in his hands, in penicillin, a material which approximated to this state of perfection. Penicillin was not, however,

Fleming's first major discovery, which instead was a substance called lysozyme. At the time of its discovery, lysozyme, like penicillin, was largely ignored, because, while it could lyse a bacterium, the organism involved was of no medical importance whatsoever. Had Fleming not discovered penicillin, then his place in the history of microbiology would have been assured by his lysozyme work..

The way in which Fleming discovered lysozyme has some startling parallels with how he came to discover penicillin, so much so that the first discovery could almost be regarded as a dress rehearsal for the more famous discovery of penicillin. Dr V. D. Allison, a young Belfast graduate, was working with Fleming in the Inoculation Department at St Mary's in 1921 when the discovery was made. Discarding some bacteriological plates one evening Fleming examined one for a while and then exclaimed 'This looks interesting.'

The plate was one on which he had begun culturing some mucus from his nose some two weeks earlier, while suffering from a head cold. What interested Fleming was that in the vicinity of this mucus a golden yellow bacterium, a contaminant from the laboratory air, was showing clear signs of being lysed. Obviously something was diffusing from the mucus and destroying the bacteria in the immediate vicinity, while lysing those further away. The parallels between this discovery and that of penicillin are obviously amazing, the main difference being that, in this case, rather than providing the source of the inhibitory agent, as in the penicillin phenomenon, the contaminant itself was being acted upon by what was growing on the plate.

Fleming next tested some fresh mucus on the bacterium and found, to his evident surprise, that within two minutes the bacterium under test was lysed so that it became as clear as water. Beginning on 23 November, Fleming then began studying the newly observed lytic phenomenon in more detail. He found that the agent responsible could be found in samples taken from all his friends and colleagues, so his own mucus was in no way special. Next, he tested other body secretions, and found that the lytic principle was widely distributed around the body and could be found in tears, saliva, sputum, blood serum, plasma and pus. In fact Fleming had made two discoveries, since the bacterium which was lysed by the lytic agent was also new to science. Realizing that the new substance would need a name, Fleming turned to Almroth Wright for help. Wright was well known as a classical scholar and keen debater; he was also fond of giving relatively simple ideas complex, mythological-sounding names. Fortunately, in this case, by suggesting that Fleming should call the lytic agent lysozyme, he hit on the perfect, succinct term which is still in use today.

Fleming's excitement at this discovery was soon to take a severe knock when he found that while the lytic phenomenon was widely distributed in body fluids of humans and other animals, its effect was limited to his own unusual bacterial contaminant (which he designated *A. F. coccus*, but was later to be named *Micrococcus lysodeikticus*). It turned out that pathogenic bacteria, such as staphylococci and streptococci, were totally unaffected by lysozyme. Fleming's dream that at last he might have found a means of treating bacterial infections was once again cruelly dashed.

Despite this obvious setback, Fleming and Allison continued to study some of the properties of lysozyme, and their results convinced Fleming that lysozyme was a 'ferment', that is, what we would now refer to as an enzyme.

In December 1921, Fleming reported his findings on lysozyme to a meeting of the Medical Research Club. He apparently showed little enthusiasm for his discovery and at the end of his talk the audience asked no questions. As far as they were concerned, here was some rare and harmless germ which was lysed by body fluids. The discovery had no possible use in medicine; it was the first of 'Flem's foolish whims'.

Interestingly, Fleming does not appear to have been the first person to report the fact that tears had a bactericidal action. As long ago as 1889, a Frenchman called Valude claimed in the journal *Annales d'Ocultistique* that 'tears could destroy the virulence of the anthrax bacillus, the colon bacillus and the yellow staphylococcus.' Whatever Valude was working with, it clearly was not lysozyme, and one cannot imagine that if such a substance, capable of such a wide antibacterial effect, were present in tears it would not have been more widely studied, and perhaps used in therapy. Similarly, as early as 1893, Wurt and Lermoyez reported that nasal mucus has bactericidal properties, but again the claims which they made for its widespread inhibitory action prove that they must have been working with something other than lysozyme.

In 1972, the proceedings of a conference to commemorate Fleming's discovery of lysozyme included reference to some 2,586 papers devoted to this single substance! Once again, Fleming's gift for making important discoveries had confounded the critics.

One of the first people, other than Fleming, to take an interest in lysozyme was Howard Florey. Florey's first collaborator in this work was Neil Goldsworthy, who was given the task of determining the lysozyme content of a whole range of animal secretions. Fleming provided Florey with a culture of *M. lysodeikticus*, the susceptible test bacterium, and Goldsworthy employed Fleming's methods to learn more about the properties of this mysterious new lytic agent.

Florey continued to take an interest in lysozyme throughout the 1930s and, in 1936, Ernst Chain and a research student called Leslie Epstein began a programme of work aimed at further studying lysozyme and isolating it in the pure form. They were to show that lysozyme is an enzyme which destroys a polysaccharide called N-acetyl glucosamine which is present in the cell walls of *M. lysodeikticus*.

With the problem of the nature of lysozyme neatly solved Chain found himself at something of a loose end. The perhaps obvious next step was to investigate other antimicrobial products found in nature, a decision which, as we have seen, was to lead Florey and Chain to begin their momentous studies of Fleming's second major discovery, penicillin.

MICROBIAL ANTAGONISM TO ANTIBIOTICS

From the earliest days of microbiology, certain microorganisms were observed to inhibit the growth of others, and, as we have seen, such studies have often been misinterpreted as being early discoveries of penicillin. A remarkable accidental observation, one of the many to occur in the history of antibiotics, convinced Pasteur of the powerful potential of microbial antagonism. He was in the process of growing the anthrax bacillus on urine when he noticed that his culture had become contaminated. Rather than throw it away, he kept it overnight. When he returned next day he found that the anthrax bacillus had been completely destroyed by the invader. Although Pasteur immediately recognized the potential use of this antagonism in medicine, his experiments on the effect proved to be uncharacteristically haphazard. Instead of isolating the organism which was responsible for killing the pathogen, as Fleming was later to do, Pasteur merely injected a guinea pig with a dose of the anthrax bacillus and followed it with injections of isolations of various airborne microorganisms. Needless to say, the results were disappointing. Pasteur had, however, established the provocative idea that microorganisms might be pitted against one another in the battle against infection.

By the late 1880s, all manner of observations on microbial antagonism were being made and attempts were underway to employ the phenomenon against pathogenic bacteria. In 1888, Max Bierfreund was working on rigor mortis in the Physiology Institute of Korngsberg in Russia. He described what he saw as follows: 'Mould fungi which flourish excellently on acid medium appeared on the muscles on the second day and multiplied so rapidly that the muscles were soon enveloped as by a white mantle. The mould fungi, in their turn, have prevented the development of putrid organisms [i.e. bacteria].' In 1885 he suggested: 'If the study of mutual antagonisms of bacteria were sufficiently far advanced, a disease caused by one bacterium probably could be treated by another. A further and wider study of this reciprocal action of bacteria may lead to new ideas in therapeutics.' Then, in the same year, Cantani put this theory to practical test, when he treated a 4-year old girl suffering from tuberculosis with a bronchial insufflation of a nonpathogenic bacterium, *Bacillus thermophilus* . At the end of a 26-day treatment period, he claimed that the tubercle bacillus was no longer present in the girl's sputum and that she had been cured.

Cantani's work was then followed by one of the most remarkable early uses of a microbial metabolite when Rudolph Emmerich and Oscar Low showed that the culture filtrates of *Bacillus pyocyaneus* (now *Pseudomonas aeruginosa*) could kill a variety of pathogenic bacteria, and even nullify the effects of the diphtheria toxin. Animal tests confirmed the effectiveness of this new substance which was called pyocyanase. By 1901, a reasonably pure form of pyocyanase was being produced on a commercial scale throughout the countries of continental Europe. Pyocyanase was generally used on surface infections, but on occasions it was also given intravenously and even injected into the spine. A variety of modifications of the basic substance appeared, beginning in 1910, with pyocyaneine, a preparation introduced by Fortineau, which was made by extracting a culture of *B. pyocyaneus* with ether.

Before long, however, tests with pyocyanase began to reveal strange inconsistencies in its effectiveness. While on some occasions it would cure infections, on others it would appear totally useless. Not surprisingly, doctors soon tired of this variability, and pyocyanase was eventually abandoned to go the way of many other potentially promising antibacterial agents.

However, despite the failure of pyocyanase, researchers continued to examine examples of microbial antagonism for possible cures. In 1907, for example, Maurice Nicolle sampled the earth of Constantinople and from it extracted a strain of *Bacillus subtilis* which he claimed was capable of lysing the typhoid bacillus. Unfortunately it also had the undesirable effect of lysing the red blood corpuscles and so was quickly abandoned! By 1919, Albert Vaudremer had reported that the fungus *Aspergillus fumigatus* could attenuate the tubercle bacillus, but once again the effect seems to have been very variable and it was not pursued.

The ability of actinomycetes to antagonize fungi and other bacteria was also frequently observed prior to the initiation of screening programmes by Waksman and associates at Rutgers in the early 1940s. In 1923, for example, Andre Gratia and Maurice Welsch showed that culture filtrates from these organisms could lyse bacteria. Some of the most thorough of these studies were carried out by a German bacteriologist, Rudolf Lieske. Lieske wrote a book in 1921, called *The Morphology and Biology of the* Streptomyces,' in which he described how *Streptomyces* species cause the lysis and death of bacteria when growing on agar plates. Lieske concluded that 'whether the bacteriolytic *enzyme* [my italics] of the actinomycetes could ever be of therapeutic value is questionable, but not completely unlikely.' In a paper which he wrote in 1949 Lieske emphasized that a considerable amount of work had been done on the antibacterial activity of actinomycetes long before Waksman's work, and that strains possessing this ability could be readily obtained from a culture collection in Baarn, Holland. Needless to say, despite this fact, it was not until Waksman's work that actinomycete antibiotics became widely available for medical use.

At the beginning of this century, microbiologists turned their attentions to the question of what happens to pathogenic bacteria when their victims are buried, in particular whether or not the bodies act as reservoirs of infection. During these studies further examples of microbial antagonism were observed. For example, Dr Sydney Martin in the Supplement to the *13th Annual Report Of the Medical Office of the English Local Government Board for 1900–1901* reported the following: 'The disappearance of typhoid bacillus is not due to their requiring and using all the organic matter in the soil, but seems to be the result of the poisonous effect of the soil microorganisms on the typhoid bacillus.'

It is clear then that microbial antagonism was widely studied both in the laboratory and in the environment, where it was thought to have a major influence on the ecology of microbial populations. The ability of microorganisms, particularly fungi, to antagonize the growth of others continued to be observed right up until the eve of the antibiotic era. Edwin C. White, for example, while working at the Johns Hopkins Hospital reported that *Aspergillus flavus* yielded filtrates which were inhibitory to both Gram-positive and Gram-negative bacteria. This work was published in the eminent journal *Science* on 9 August 1940, just as Florey and the Oxford group were preparing their first paper on penicillin. One can only assume that with some trepidation one of their number rushed to the nearest library to look up White's report. The title of this paper, 'Bactericidal Filtrate from a Mould Culture', must have momentarily made the individual members of the Oxford team miss a heartbeat and fear that someone had got to penicillin ahead of them!

The appearance of purified penicillin and then of antibiotics like streptomycin must have made those microbiologists who had observed the phenomenon of microbial antagonism, but had failed to act, sorely rue their missed opportunity. A number of such sorry tales can be found in the scientific literature. In a recent obituary of the US mycologist, Walter Henry Snell, for example, it was said that 'he had made observations on antibiotic producing fungi prior to Fleming's publication, but an assistant cleaned up the cultures before the work could be published.' In a similar vein, a certain T. Lishman wrote to the *Veterinary Record* in 1947, describing how in the early 1900s Professor M'Fadyean introduced students to bacteriology classes at the Royal Veterinary College by urging upon them the necessity of covering up as early as possible tubes and petri dishes inoculated with organisms which they wished to incubate. He then apparently picked up a petri dish which had long been in the incubator, removed the cover and said:

> Look at this as a warning against delay. I inoculated this medium with a loop of material containing staphylococci, but before I could place the cover over the Petri dish a spore of some kind of fungus floating about in the air alighted upon the culture medium. It will be noticed that while some of the colonies of staphylococci have grown, the growth from this spore of a parasitic fungus, apparently akin to the ordinary common mould, has also flourished and it will be further noticed that the growth of this fungus has had a marked deleterious effect on the growth of the staphylococci, either owing to exhalation of something, or addition of something to the culture medium, which has been decidedly inimical to the colonies of staphylococci. In fact the growth of the colonies immediately adjacent to the fungoid growth appears to have been completely inhibited. The only thing to do now is to throw the culture away.

Lishman concludes his letter with the words: 'How near was our greatest teacher to making what has since become a world famous discovery?' Very near, perhaps, but the difference between a keen observer, such as his former professor, and a person who achieves immortality is possession of 'the prepared mind' and the will to act, characteristics which clearly distinguished Fleming from his less fortunate predecessors.

Besredka's Antivirus

During the early part of this century, a French scientist called Besredka, while working at the Pasteur Institute, developed an unusual approach to the treatment of bacterial infection, which came to be called Besredka's antivirus. Besredka was born in Odessa, Russia in 1870, and had followed Metchnikoff to the Pasteur Institute. When Metchnikoff died, Besredka assumed the role of Director of the Institute and, until his death in 1940, he made a number of important contributions to the sciences of bacteriology and immunology.

The modern reader might assume that the term 'antivirus' would refer to a treatment for viral infections, such as the common cold or AIDS. In fact, Besredka claimed that his antivirus was effective in the treatment of bacterial infections. The antivirus principle was widely used in the treatment of disease; it had an important impact on the way Fleming came to regard the nature of penicillin and as a result on the history of medicine as a whole.

Antivirus therapy involved the application to wounds or surface infections of a filtered broth on which a bacterium had been grown to exhaustion. The broth contained the antivirus, which was said to be specific; that is, a medium which, for example, had nurtured *Staphylococcus* was only effective when used to treat infections caused by this bacterium, but would have no effect on an infection caused by a *Streptococcus*. It is important to stress that Besredka did not regard his antivirus as being representative of an inhibitor which we would now refer to as being an antibiotic. He thought that the antivirus acted by stimulating the patient's own immunity rather than by directly killing the bacterium which caused the infection.

Although Besredka's antivirus was widely used especially on the Continent, it was not without its critics. Even some of his advocates maintained that it was unnecessary to grow a specific bacterium on the broth, since they claimed that uncontaminated but filtered broth would achieve the same curative effect. A large number of reports appeared in the medical literature of the 1930s claiming to demonstrate the effectiveness of the antivirus therapy against a wide range of bacterial infections. However, since the treatment was never exposed to the rigours of a clinical trial, we can never be certain of just how effective it was. Antivirus was produced on a commercial scale, both in England and on the Continent. Doctors could obtain a proprietary product or have a large supply of antivirus prepared from one of their own isolates.

An excellent example of the kind of cures which are said to have been achieved by the use of this therapy was reported by two US doctors,

Merten and Oesterlin, in 1932. They described how a 12-year old boy had broken his arm in a fall from a tree. On arrival at the Milwaukee Hospital his radius was protruding some two and a half inches from out of his right arm. The fracture was operated on and a splint was applied. Some four weeks after the accident, and despite extensive conventional treatment, the wound became infected with *Clostridium* and gas gangrene developed. On the twenty-eighth day of his confinement in hospital, Oesterlin prepared an antivirus produced from a wound isolate. This was then applied to the infection using a soaked dressing. At first, the boy's temperature rose but then it fell again to normal. Merten and Oesterlin claimed a cure, and concluded that without treatment the boy would definitely have lost his arm.

Besredka's antivirus theories were greeted with considerable scepticism in Britain. It is not surprising, therefore, that when his ideas were related by a colleague, Dr Broughton Alcock, to a meeting of the Royal Society of Medicine on 15 May 1929, they were met with a less than sympathetic hearing. The lecture's content was severely criticized, both by those in attendance and the medical press.

One of the members of the audience at that meeting was none other than Alexander Fleming, and he rose at the end to give his impression of the validity of Besredka's treatment. There is no doubt that, like most of the other scientists who attended that meeting, Fleming was initially sceptical about the concept. He compared antivirus with penicillin, explaining that, like antivirus, penicillin was produced by growing an organism, in this case a mould, in broth culture. Fleming then went on to describe his first attempts to use crude penicillin to treat a case of indolent ulcer of the leg (presumably with the help of Dickson Wright). Fleming clearly did not believe at this point that penicillin acted in the way claimed for antivirus, that is, by inducing a local immunity. Instead, he obviously thought that its curative effects directly resulted from its ability to kill the offending pathogenic bacterium.

However, by 1931, Fleming seems to have changed his mind about the nature of penicillin, since in his second paper on the subject he states that 'It is unlikely that penicillin acts by killing bacteria directly'. He then continues with the following remarkable statement: 'Gratia and others have shown that when compresses of broth are applied to the skin there is an aggregation of phagocytic cells in the deeper layers and he has thus explained the rationale of Besredka's antivirus treatment. Penicillin might act in the same way as antivirus but superior to ordinary *antivirus* [my italics] in that it inhibits the growth of not only one but all pyogenic bacteria.' It is possible that Fleming's new-found views on the way penicillin acts are not as far-fetched as they may at first sight appear. We have already noted that in the 1940s scientists found that partially purified extracts of penicillin seemed to be more effective as a chemotherapeutic agent than pure penicillin. Dr J. Ungar, for example, while working at the Glaxo Laboratories in Greenford, Middlesex, reported in the *British Medical Journal* in 1949 that the 'enhancement' effect of impure penicillin was due to the activation of certain defence mechanisms, rather than to any direct action of any impurities on penicillin itself. It seems that Fleming, because of his fondness for performing counts of white blood cells, came to discover this secondary enhancement effect, and it was these observations which caused him to change his mind about the nature of penicillin.

By 1931 then, Fleming had clearly come to believe that penicillin stimulated the host's immunity to infection, as well as directly killing bacteria. He began to see it as a form of antivirus. As a result, anyone reading Fleming's second paper would have assumed that penicillin was just another antivirus, the concept of which had been largely discredited. Add this fact to penicillin's notorious instability, and there was every reason why it should have been ignored.

BACTERIOPHAGE THERAPY: THE CLINICAL USE OF 'VIRAL ANTIBIOTICS'

Yet another interesting approach to the cure of bacterial infections which was quite extensively evaluated prior to the advent of the chemotherapeutic age involved the use of bacteriophage. These are viruses which prey on bacteria, including pathogens. They were first described in 1915 by the English bacteriologist, Frederick Twort. The same phenomenon was then independently discovered two years later by Felix d'Herelle of the Pasteur Institute, and, as a result, the ability of certain viruses to lyse bacteria is often referred to as the 'Twort-d'Herelle phenomenon'. Since bacteriophages have the ability to infect bacteria and cause them to burst and then die, it was not long after their discovery that the possibility was suggested of using them to cure bacterial infections. In fact, although Twort first suggested this possibility, it was d'Herelle who was to become the chief exponent of the practical use of bacteriophage in therapy. In 1927, while in India, d'Herelle attempted to use bacteriophage to treat Asiatic cholera. The phage was given to patients in spoonfuls while patients for whom it was denied acted as controls. D'Herelle claimed that the treatment was a success, with mortality rates in the treated group being around 8 per cent, compared to over 60 per cent mortality amongst the controls.

Bacteriophage therapy appeared most successful when it was used to treat surface problems, although it was also applied to the intestinal lumen, nasal sinuses and in the treatment of urinary tract infections. More surprisingly, however, attempts were even made to inject bacteriophage into the blood stream, despite the well-known fact that blood, pus and antiseptics tended to inhibit bacteriophage action. It seems that bacteriophage therapy was particularly useful in the treatment of boils and carbuncles, when the phage was introduced into the lymph space about the boil through a very fine needle. In 1932, Dr J. Ward MacNeal of the New York Hospital recommended this technique for routine use for treating infections caused by staphylococci, so it appears to have been relatively successful. Infected wounds could also be treated by applying dressings wet with staphylococcal broth bacteriophage filtrate in a manner not unlike that used in Besredka's antivirus therapy. During the early 1930s, approaches like antivirus, bacteriophage therapy and maggot therapy (which will be discussed below) must have vied with one another for the accolade of the most effective available treatment for bacterial infections.

One of the problems which must have militated against the effectiveness of this therapy was the common belief that bacteriophage was a single agent. This is not the case, however, as bacteriophages are specific to certain bacteria, such that staphylococcal bacteriophages, for example, will only lyse and kill staphylococci and related bacteria. Bacteriophage was not therefore a general antiseptic, since it was essential that the bacterium involved in the infection be identified and a specific bacteriophage developed and employed against the infection it caused. It is possible that where bacteriophages were effective the result was due to the fact that phage filtrates may act as specific vaccines, since they contain the antigens of lysed bacteria, or alternatively as stimulants of a nonspecific immunity.

Despite the many and varied claims for the success of bacteriophage, it is now generally accepted that only in exceptional circumstances has phage any *in vivo* antibacterial action. Some recent studies may, however, require a reappraisal of this orthodox view. The most exciting claims for the successful use of bacteriophage therapy have been reported from Poland, by Dr Stephen Slopek and colleagues at the Polish Academy of Science's Institute of Immunology and Experimental Therapy. In these studies, bacteriophage was given by mouth or applied directly to wounds. In 121 of the patients the infections were cured completely while some improvements were shown in the remaining 7. What is particularly interesting about this work is that the infections were caused by bacteria which were resistant to conventional antibiotics. Interestingly, in 1945, a certain F. Himmelweit worked under Fleming's guidance at St Mary's on the possibility that penicillin and bacteriophage might have a combined action on staphylococci. The combination seemed appropriate because both agents are known to lyse these bacteria. The results of this work, published in the *Lancet*, showed that penicillin did not affect the multiplication of the *Staphylococcus* bacteriophage nor did it interfere with its lethal and lytic action. Himmelweit also showed that a mixture of penicillin and phage could kill bacteria even when they were resistant to the action of the antibiotic.

It has been argued that the development of bacteriophage-resistant bacteria is unlikely, and this fact, together with the specificity, cheapness and apparent total lack of associated side effects, have tempted some to suggest that we are on the verge of a new approach to the treatment of bacterial infections. It is highly unlikely, however, that Selman Waksman would have approved of the term 'viral antibiotics' to describe this approach.

MAGGOT THERAPY: A BIZARRE INTERLUDE IN THE STORY OF ANTIBIOTICS

Before the appearance of the sulphonamides and then penicillin, there was little that doctors could do to treat long-standing bacterial infections. The frustration that they felt in the face of such impotence is not difficult to imagine, and it is perhaps not surprising to learn that some of them turned to what must be the most bizarre form of antibacterial treatment, maggot therapy. As its name suggests, this involved the use of live maggots to treat infections! Surprisingly, this therapy was not quackery, but a serious and systematic attempt to cure a range of bacterial infections.

Maggot therapy proved to be particularly successful in the treatment of a distressing disease common amongst children, called osteomyelitis. This bacterial infection of the long bones, for which there was no cure in the early thirties, was eventually defeated first by the sulphonamides and then by penicillin. Prior to their appearance, however, maggot therapy proved the only effective treatment for osteomyelitis and many other infections caused by bacteria. How did this repellent approach to curing bacterial infections ever become established in the medical repertoire?

The answer is that, like so many other developments in medicine, maggot therapy did not originate as a rational attempt to treat disease, but instead evolved from a wide variety of observations stretching back into antiquity. For centuries past, military surgeons had observed that the wounds of soldiers left on the battlefield were often found to be in better condition than if they had been taken directly to a field hospital and then treated with antiseptics. The surprisingly healthy condition of these wounds was often found to be due to the presence of live maggots. It seemed that maggots fed on the dying flesh, removing debris and thereby promoting healthy tissue granulation.

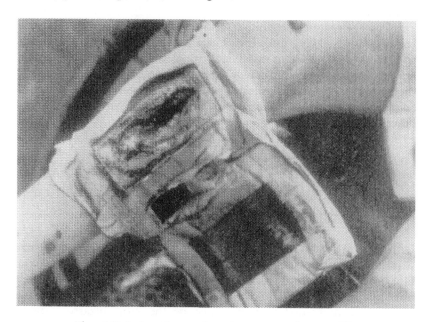

Plate 10(a) A patient undergoing maggot therapy. The cage was used to contain the live maggots within the wound

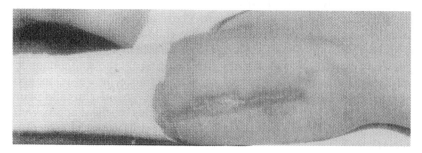

Plate 10(b) A case of tuberculosis hip cured using maggot therapy

The beneficial action of maggots on wounds had been observed by the surgeon Ambrose Pare after the battle of St Quentin in 1557, and similar observations were made by Baron De Jong during the Napoleonic Wars. More recently, the beneficial effects of maggots on the wounds of battle casualties was seen in the American Civil and First World Wars, and even used by American prisoners during the Korean War. An example of the use of this therapy in military medicine was described by a Confederate physician, J. F. Zacharias, as follows:

> During my services at Danville, Virginia, I first used maggots to remove the decayed tissue in hospital gangrene and with eminent satisfaction. In a single day they would clean a wound much better than any agents we had in our command. I used them afterwards at various places. I am sure I saved many lives by their use, escaped septicaemia, and had rapid recoveries.

However, despite the numerous historical references to the beneficial effects of maggots on wounds, they appear to have been rarely used in civilian medicine, until a US surgeon, William S. Baer, began using them in his clinical practice to treat osteomyelitis. Despite the fact that Baer is usually credited with being the first person to introduce maggot therapy into civilian practice, the following letter by Dr R. F. Kampmeier, which appeared in 1987 in the *Southern Medical Journal*, suggests that the therapy was in common use before Baer's work:

> Several years ago, in writing an autobiography for my family, I made note of the following experiences in my years as a rotating intern in Salt Lake City Hospital (1923–1924). I recall patients with chronic osteomyelitis, the bane of hospitals in those days, who in addition to saucerization, had an unusual treatment. Dr Pugh, who had had experience on the Western Front in World War One, would upon occasion telegraph for sterile maggots which arrived in special containers. We would apply maggots in some instances of chronic osteomyelitis or infected compound fractures, and they really cleaned up the necrotic tissue so fresh granulation tissue might form. When one wished to sterilize the wound of maggots one merely poured in ether.

William Stevenson Baer was born in Baltimore in 1872. He graduated from Johns Hopkins University in 1894, and after obtaining his MD, became a surgeon at his Alma Mater, finally reaching the status of the

First Clinical Assistant of Orthopaedic Surgery in 1917. Baer was also influential in the creation of the Children's Hospital in Baltimore. In championing maggot therapy Baer was therefore risking an orthodox and highly successful medical career. However, he had seen the surprising effects of maggots on infected wounds while surviving in France during the First World War, so he was determined that on his return to civilian life he would try and evaluate the applicability of the technique to general practice.

It has been estimated that when Baer began using maggot therapy in 1930 there were some 10,000 unhealed cases of osteomyelitis in the US alone. This disease is characterized by inflammation of the long bones, which eventually leads to bone destruction, unhealed wounds and deformity. Prior to the appearance of the sulphonamides and penicillin, wounds caused by this infection would often remain infected for long periods, breaking down periodically over many years and necessitating frequent operations. Before the introduction of maggot therapy the only hope of treating these wounds was to flood them with antiseptics, an approach which usually failed.

The maggots used in this approach to therapy were not the blue blowflies used by fishermen, but the closely related green blowfly or *Lucilia sericata*. In fact, members of the genus *Lucilia* were so widely used to treat infected wounds that they became known as surgical maggots. Doctors generally reared their own supplies of maggots, although they could also buy them from commercial supply houses. This would have proved prohibitive in most cases, however, as the cost, at today's prices, of treating a single patient would approach 1,000 dollars! The maggots were generally reared from eggs, and fed on a mixture of pig's liver and yeast extract. They were kept in a refrigerator to reduce their activity until required. Baer originally suggested that maggots should be sterilized before use so as to avoid the possibility of them transmitting tetanus (i.e. lockjaw) to patients. However, this costly and time-consuming step was later avoided by administering precautionary anti-tetanus injections.

The technique employed by Baer involved placing maggots inside the open wound and preventing their escape by strapping a cage to the infected limb. An electric light bulb was often suspended over the cage, forcing the maggots to go deep into the wound to seek shade. Here they would clean the bone and remove dead flesh without attacking living material. Every practitioner of maggot therapy had their own tricks. For example, some recommended that vaseline be smeared around the wound so that any maggot that tried to escape would slip and fall back in! The psychological effects of this treatment on the patients involved, particularly children, can only be imagined. The physical effects seem bad enough, ranging from a slight tickling sensation to searing pain which could only be relieved with morphine.

Baer believed that the curative effects of maggot therapy were more complex than merely their ability to clean the wound and that they produced antibacterial as well as wound-healing secretions. This raised the hope that if such secretions could be isolated then the unpleasant aspect of using live maggots could be avoided. The British medical bacteriologist, L. P. Garrod, was less than convinced, however. In 1935, he wrote: 'The idea of using excrement as an antiseptic is so novel, not to say fantastic, that it must command interest and good wishes to anyone who out of the strangest and most repulsive therapeutic innovation of recent times has been able to extract an idea which is stranger still.' Nevertheless, researchers during the 1930s continued to make a frantic search for this miracle ingredient responsible for the effectiveness of maggot therapy. At first it was suggested that allantoin or urea were responsible for the healing and antibacterial action of maggot secretions. Then attention turned to ammonia, a breakdown product of urea. In fact the active ingredient was never to be found during the time when this technique was in use, and as a result live maggots had to be employed right up until the point when the sulphonamides took over from this gruesome treatment. However, S. W. Simmons of the US Bureau of Entomology showed in 1935 that maggot washings contained compounds which could kill the bacteria which cause wound infections. His paper ends with this remarkably prophetic statement: 'From the tests described herein it is the author's belief that intensive investigations of bactericidal substances produced by living organisms is a fertile field in which new substances may perhaps be isolated to cope with situations which do not yield to ordinary antiseptics.' It is likely, however, that Simmons was thinking here of substances produced by higher organisms, rather than bacteria and fungi, so while he foresaw the antibiotic era, his views on the likely source of the antibiotics was perhaps somewhat off target.

Simmons's work was not to represent the last attempt to find the curative agent present in maggot washings. As late as 1957, two English scientists, E. R. Pavillard and E. P. Wright, ironically while working at St Mary's Hospital, concluded that the active ingredient involved in maggot therapy was a fatty acid. Samples of their extracts were sent to Porton Down, then a defence research establishment, for further study. Although the extracts were analysed, the results were never released, for the somewhat surprising, if not alarming, reason that they contained compounds which were included on Porton's classified list!

The most recent attempt to explain the effectiveness of maggot therapy was made by a US team led by G. R. Erdmann. They concluded that maggot secretions harbour a bacterium, called *Proteus mirabilis*, which produces two antibacterial compounds, phenylacetic acid and phenylacetaldehyde.

We should perhaps not be too complacent about seeing the last of this repulsive therapy, since the technique was recently used with success to treat a wound infected with antibiotic-resistant bacteria. This case was reported in June 1976 by a team of doctors at the University of Texas Health Science Centre, led by Karl Lawrence Horn. They described in the journal *Archives of Otorhinolaryngology* how they treated a 67-year old man suffering from mastoiditis (a complication of a middle ear infection, where the infection spreads to the mastoid bone behind the ear, causing pain and also possibly deafness and even meningitis) which had been brought about by wearing a hearing aid. The infection had been caused by the bacteria *Pseudomonas* sp., *Proteus mirabilis* and species of *Enterococcus*. Conventional antibiotic therapy failed and the doctors were forced to employ maggot therapy. The maggots were introduced into the mastoid cavity behind the ear, and two weeks later the patient was discharged. The paper describing this case concluded as follows:

> The intractable nature of this man's infection makes it clear that without maggot therapy healing would not have occurred. The authors recognize that this unusual form of therapy is not part of the standard armamentarium against infections of the temporal bone. We see no need to categorically discard successful techniques of the past, however, because one never knows when they might be useful in the future. We feel justified in using this otherwise antiquated technique in a situation in which modern technology was inadequate.

Maggot washings have also recently been evaluated in the treatment of extensive burns. Leeches, too, have recently made a comeback into medicine. Perhaps we have not yet seen the last of maggot therapy!

BACTERIAL PRODUCTS IN THE TREATMENT OF CANCER

In the last chapter, we will discover that some established antibiotics are currently in use to help in the treatment of cancers, while newly discovered compounds continue to be evaluated for this purpose. Such usage obviously falls into the realm of 'scientific medicine', and is clearly regarded as being acceptable in the eyes of the medical-scientific community. In this section, however, I wish to discuss a form of anti-cancer treatment involving the use of bacterial vaccines which, although long established, remains far more speculative than cancer drug therapy.

In 1891, a young New York surgeon called William B. Coley lost his first case of cancer, a woman of 19, who died despite early radical surgery for a sarcoma. Coley recognized that surgery alone was not the answer to cancer treatment, so he began looking through the records of about 100 cancer patients in the hope of finding a clue to a more acceptable and effective form of treatment. His researches brought him to the amazing realization that when cancer patients simultaneously suffered from a bacterial infection, such as erysepalis, then they stood a better chance of recovery from the tumour than in the absence of the infection. This led Coley to try and induce erysepalis in inoperable cases of cancer. This proved unsuccessful, so next he tried treatment with a mixed filtered vaccine made from streptococci, and the toxins of *Bacillus prodigiosus* (now *Serratia marcescens*). The first case to receive this mixed filterable vaccine was a bedridden 19-year old man, with an inoperable sarcoma of the abdominal wall and pelvis. No other treatment was given, and the patient appeared cured and remained well until he suddenly died of a heart attack, some 26 years later!

The use of these Coley vaccines, as they are now called, relates to a phenomenon which has been recognized for over 200 years, namely that patients can undergo dramatic regressions of a variety of neoplastic diseases during or following a concurrent bacterial infection. As early as 1813, Vautier, for example, observed that breast cancers appeared to regress if a patient simultaneously suffered from gangrene. Then, in the mid-1800s, a Belgian scientist, Didot, put the observation that infection with syphilis appeared to cure cancer to an unorthodox and, at least by today's standards, unprincipled use. He stated that since ancient times it had been observed that prostitutes never contracted uterine cancer, while 'good, pious women' proved the most common victims. He concluded that syphilis protected the prostitutes from this form of cancer, and decided to put this theory to the test by inoculating pus from syphilic chancres from the cervix in an inoperable case of breast cancer! Symptoms of syphilis then developed, which were treated with mercury treatment, and the breast cancer diminished until the patient appeared cured.

A version of Coley's mixed vaccine was marketed by Parke Davis and company from 1889 until 1907, but it proved too weak and variable to be a success. The Lister Institute then produced a variant for the next 40 years or so. It is usually assumed, however, that it was Coley's failure to arrange a proper clinical trial to evaluate his toxins which brought about their ultimate neglect.

The use of mixed bacterial vaccines is by no means an historical oddity. There is now a considerable body of more modern data which indicates the effectiveness of this form of treatment. In 1959, for example, Huth in Germany showed that the survival rate amongst leukaemia sufferers can be improved by the use of a *Pseudomonas aeruginosa* vaccine. Over the last 40 or so years, Helen Coley Nautts and her team have assembled detailed histories of nearly 1000 cases where mixed bacterial vaccines have been useful or curative in cancer treatment. The sceptics, of which there are many, should consult the reference given to the detailed studies on this therapy given in the literature citation to this book. The reference contains many examples of scientifically based studies from orthodox cancer research institutes which point to the effectiveness of mixed vaccine therapy, evidence which seems to be ignored by many cancer specialists. The current theory which is used to account for the apparent effectiveness of such mixed bacterial vaccines is that bacteria infection induces fever, heat and inflammation which helps defeat the cancer.

Although mixed vaccine cancer therapy relies upon the use of bacterial products, it does not directly involve antibiotics. However, there is an interesting connection between the theory behind this form of treatment and today's extensive use of antibiotics. This is the view that a contributory factor to the increase in cancer might be the widespread use of antibiotics since 1940. Meyer and Benjafield suggested that 'the antibiotics may absolve the body of the need to bring the normal immunological mechanisms into use – a mechanism that has been acquired and perfected through millions of years of evolution.' This view is backed up by epidemiological data which shows that in both the developed and developing countries the incidence of infection is decreasing at the same time that cancer is increasing. We are faced with the possibility, therefore, that while the widespread use of antibiotics has led to a reduction in deaths from infectious disease it may in fact have increased fatalities due to cancers!

FALSE DAWN OF THE ANTIBIOTIC AGE

Although penicillin is generally regarded as the first antibiotic, it was in fact preceded by a compound called tyrothricin, which, while being used in medicine a few years before penicillin, proved too toxic to be injected into the blood stream, and as a result, was relegated to a minor role in the treatment of bacterial infection. It did, however, find widespread use in the treatment of surface wounds and infections. Tyrothricin and its derivatives were soon to be replaced by penicillin and the later antibiotics but had these not appeared then this compound might have been more widely used in medicine. The appearance of this antibiotic unfortunately turned out to be something of a false dawn to the antibiotic era.

Tyrothricin was discovered by Rene Dubos, a Frenchman who began his career as a scientist under the guidance of Selman Waksman. Dubos was born in 1901, in the small French village of St Brice near Paris. He graduated from the National Institute of Agronomy in Paris in 1921, but, rather than pursue a scientific career, he became the assistant editor of an agricultural journal published in Rome. It was in this city that soil scientists from all around the world met in 1924 to attend an international symposium. As with many aspects of the history of antibiotics, there are two accounts of how the young Rene was attracted to Rutgers University. In the generally related version of the story, he met Jacob Lipman at the above meeting and asked his advice. Lipman was then the Director of the New Jersey Agricultural Station at Rutgers. Seizing his opportunity, Dubos enquired of Lipman if there was any possibility that he might be taken on as a research student in his laboratory. Lipman replied that, while there was space, he had no funds to support any more graduate students. Undaunted, Dubos accepted the offer of a place, confident that he could pay his own way. In the second account, which was related by Dubos in an interview with M. Reiner in 1980, and is therefore presumably the true story, Dubos had already, and for no particular reason, decided to emigrate to the United States and he met Waksman on the boat as the Rutgers scientist was returning from the Rome conference. However, whatever the origin of the decision, it is clear that Dubos began working at Rutgers in 1924, under the supervision of Waksman rather than Lipman. Waksman, who was then establishing himself as one of the doyens of soil microbiology, suggested that Dubos should study the factors which influence the microbial breakdown of cellulose in soils, a research topic that required Dubos to become familiar with the factors which influence the activity of bacterial and fungal enzymes.

As he began this work, similar studies on enzyme activity were being conducted at the Rockefeller Institute in New York, under the direction of O. T. Avery. Avery was interested in finding a way to destroy the protective outer coat of the bacterium causing pneumonia, in the hope that it might then be susceptible to chemical attack. As Avery and Dubos had a mutual interest in polymer-degrading enzymes it is not surprising that they eventually came to work together to concentrate on solving the problem of how best to dissolve the pneumococcal coat. Dubos, with his extensive knowledge of soil microorganisms, suggested that the soil would probably be an excellent source of microorganisms which could produce cell wall lysing enzymes. As a result, he began his search by taking beakers of soil and adding pneumococcal cell walls in the hope of enriching for organisms which could degrade them. Soon an isolate was obtained which produced a cell wall lysing enzyme, able to cure artificially induced infections in mice. Unfortunately, as was too often the case, the extract proved far too toxic to be used in medicine.

Dubos eventually left Avery's laboratory, and some years later he resumed his search for antibiotic-producing soil microorganisms. Unfortunately, he concentrated his attention on isolating true bacteria, and so neglected the fungi and actinomycetes, which later proved to be the source of by far the majority of the antibiotics used in medicine.

The screening programme initiated by Dubos did produce results, however, leading to the introduction into medicine of a compound called gramicidin. This antibiotic was isolated from a strain of *Bacillus brevis*. Later, working with Rollin and Hotchkiss, Dubos isolated a crystalline substance from tyrothricin, which was given the name gramicidin, in honour of the originator of the famous bacteriological strain, Christian Gram.

While gramicidin was more effective than the sulphonamides at killing bacteria, its toxicity severely limited its use. Unfortunately, even dilute solutions of gramicidin S were shown to dissolve red blood corpuscles, and, despite a number of attempts to reduce its toxic effect, gramicidin was relegated to relative obscurity. Interestingly, a variant of gramicidin called gramicidin S was to be used throughout the war by the Soviets as their main antibiotic. It was first discovered by Dr G. F. Gause and N. Brazhnikova, who screened many hundreds of soil bacteria before isolating an antibiotic-producing strain of *Bacillus brevis*, the bacterium from which Dubos had isolated tyrothricin. Unlike penicillin, gramicidin S was too toxic for internal use, but was widely used in war surgery for the control of local infections.

Commercial preparations of gramicidin are still employed, largely as ointments in the treatment of vaginal infections, or as dusting powders for use on wounds. Tyrothricin was also used widely as an additive to throat lozenges (e.g. 'Tyrozets'), although the commercial success of these probably resulted from the small amount of pain-killing benzocaine which they contained, rather than any antibiotic effect. Gramicidin did, however, find a wider use in the treatment of mastitis in cattle.

Dubos deserves considerable credit for realizing that soil micro-organisms were a potentially rich source of antibiotic-producing microorganisms. Had he had a little more luck, then his name might have become as well known as Fleming's or Waksman's. In retrospect, however, we can see that he made the mistake of concentrating on the isolation of bacteria as potential antibiotic producers. Few of these organisms in fact produce antibiotics, although tyrothricin was to be followed by bacitracin, and then by the monobactams, compounds which act as the starting point for the production of semi-synthetic antibiotics like aztreonam.

8

Streptomycin and the Conquest of Tuberculosis

Streptomycin was the second of the major antibiotics to be discovered. Although it is effective in the treatment of a number of diseases, including certain forms of meningitis and plague, its fame lies in the fact that it provided the first effective cure for tuberculosis. Of all the infectious diseases which inflict themselves on mankind, tuberculosis, also referred to as consumption or phthisis, warrants special consideration. Common from the time of the pharoahs, throughout the Middle Ages, and until modern times, tuberculosis was until recently shockingly prevalent in all of the great cities of the world. With the aid of two drugs, isoniazid and PAS (para-aminosalicylic acid), streptomycin defeated tuberculosis and brought about the closure of the sanatoria which for so long had been the only hope for consumptives.

The first steps towards the modern treatment of tuberculosis were made by George Bodington, a Warwickshire doctor and graduate of Oxford and St Bartholomew's Hospital. During the 1880s, when Bodington first took an interest in this disease, it accounted for a fifth of the annual deaths in England. Tuberculosis sufferers were exposed to all manner of dubious treatments, including being locked in a closed room for long periods, and treated with antimony, digitalis, and bleeding by leeches. Bodington realized that, while town-dwellers often contracted tuberculosis, the disease was less common amongst country people, and he suggested that sufferers from the disease should avoid the oppressive and polluted air of the cities. Bodington's views, however, were quickly and mercilessly attacked by the eminent medical journal, the *Lancet*, and his ideas were largely ignored by his contemporaries. Developments in the treatment of tuberculosis then moved to Germany, where Peter Dettweiler established the first of the sanatoria, in which patients were exposed to fresh air, a varied diet, graded exercise and hydrotherapy.

Needless to say, the expense of this treatment limited it to the wealthy.

Many of Dettweiler's ideas were taken up and modified by the famous US pioneer of tuberculosis treatment, Edward Livingstone Trudeau. Born in 1848, Trudeau entered the College of Physicians and Surgeons in 1868. After graduating, he set up practice in New York, where he was successful until he began to suffer from sudden and inexplicable bouts of fever. When his illness was eventually diagnosed as advanced pulmonary tuberculosis he assumed that he had little time left to live, and so retired to the Adirondack Mountains of New York State. In 1882, Trudeau came across one of Dettweiler's papers and, hoping for a cure, he decided to apply his methods to his own tuberculosis. The results were so promising that Trudeau set up his own sanatorium for tuberculosis sufferers at Saranac Lake.

In the same year as Trudeau's conversion, the brilliant German bacteriologist, Robert Koch, discovered the tubercle bacillus, which is now referred to as *Mycobacterium tuberculosis*. Rumours then began to circulate around Germany that he had found a cure for tuberculosis. When it was announced that the Tenth International Medical Congress would be held in Berlin in the summer of 1890, it was expected that Koch would announce some major breakthrough in the treatment of tuberculosis. He was then put under immense pressure, being led to believe that the whole of Germany, including the Kaiser himself, expected great things from him, which would further emphasize the supremacy of Germanic science. The cream of the world's scientists, some 7,000 delegates, packed into the auditorium. The air of expectancy was almost unbearable. After a preamble, Koch announced that: 'I have at last hit upon a substance that has the power of preventing the growth of tubercle bacilli not only in the test tube, but in the body of an animal.' His treatment was based on the idea that tuberculosis could be cured by giving patients injections of a glycerine extract of the tubercle bacillus, an extract which Koch termed 'tuberculin'.

The response to the announcement was so overwhelming that few bothered to listen to Koch's cautious words that followed. His scientific reputation was such that a mere hint of a cure was sufficient to convince most people that at last tuberculosis was about to be defeated. Later that year Koch published the results of his apparently successful trials with tuberculin. The response amongst tuberculosis sufferers and their families was staggering. They swarmed into Berlin, and the demand for the new curative could not possibly be met. The price of tuberculin inflated dramatically, and the inevitable black market sprang up. Even Joseph Lister, the father of antiseptic surgery, was happy to see his niece exposed to Koch's treatment without ever seriously questioning its efficacy. Then tragedy struck when patients who had received the extract, including Lister's niece, began to die. In January 1891, the eminent pathologist Rudolf Virchow produced evidence to show that the corpses of 21 patients who had received tuberculin were riddled with miliary tuberculosis, the most virulent form of the disease. It was clear that the so-called treatment was actually spreading the infection! There was uproar. Koch's reputation lay in shreds, and he was even accused of being a charlatan. He was never to recover from what became known as the 'tuberculin fiasco.'

Trudeau was one of the first to recognize the dangers inherent in Koch's methods, and their failure renewed his faith in the value of sanatorium treatment. For the next 50 or so years, tuberculosis sufferers had to depend upon this form of treatment for their only real hope of a remission from the disease, and by the early 1940s there were 600 such establishments in the US alone. Other patients, like D. H. Lawrence, were advised to seek the dry air of a hot climate. For the majority, however, there was neither cure nor respite, only the reality of being condemned to a lingering and generally painful death.

Tuberculosis reached its peak at the beginning of the industrial revolution when its spread was encouraged by mass migrations from rural areas and by the overcrowded conditions developed as a result. By 1780 the mortality rate in England from this one disease was over 1,000 per 100,000 of the population, a figure which is placed in perspective by the fact that in 1930, for example, this same rate of mortality resulted from all the fatal diseases put together! By 1937, tuberculosis was the most common cause of death in the USA. The lack of immunity to this disease amongst the native Americans of the Canadian Northwest was particularly tragic; crowded into reservations, they soon fell prey to tuberculosis, so that by 1912, the mortality rate amongst these people from this one disease reached a staggering 10 per cent.

Tuberculosis sufferers received the news of the triumph which penicillin had achieved in defeating bacterial infection with great excitement. Not unnaturally, they assumed that the new wonder drug would bring an end to their suffering. However, penicillin proved to have no effect whatsoever on the tubercle bacillus. Nonetheless, the appearance of penicillin did suggest the possibility that a new antibiotic might be found which was capable of curing tuberculosis. Then, during the early 1940s, news began to leak out of a new antibiotic, called streptomycin, which might be able to cure the age-old scourge of tuberculosis.

Nearly every account of the discovery of streptomycin gives full credit for its discovery to one man, Selman Abraham Waksman. As we shall see, however, Waksman was only one of two co-discoverers of streptomycin and the involvement of the other, Albert Schatz, has remained largely ignored over the 50 years or so since the antibiotic was discovered. The story of the birth of streptomycin is no less fascinating than the penicillin story, yet relatively few accounts have appeared which detail how the world's second major antibiotic came into being. Most of the accounts of this story that have appeared were written by Waksman and, for reasons which will soon become apparent, he hardly ever referred to the role of Albert Schatz.

By the time Selman Waksman came to take a determined interest in the subject of microbial antagonism, he was already one of the world's leading soil microbiologists. He was born in 1888, in Russia. Because of anti-Semitism, Waksman was denied the opportunity of a university education, and, as a result, he emigrated to the US, arriving in 1910. After initially supporting himself by working on his cousin's farm, he enrolled at the University of New Jersey at Rutgers where he obtained a BSc. and a Master's degree. Then, after a short period in California, he returned to Rutgers to take up the post of lecturer in his old department. In the late 1930s, Waksman became interested in the subject of microbial antagonism, not from a medical standpoint, but from his desire to know more about how microorganisms interact with one another in soils.

When Waksman heard of the Oxford group's success in purifying penicillin, he is said to have exclaimed: 'Drop everything; see what these English have done with a mould. I know the actinomycetes will do better.' Waksman was, in fact, one of the few people up to that point to have taken an interest in the ecology and physiology of the soil actinomycetes. Now he saw the opportunity of using this knowledge to begin a screening programme which he felt sure would lead to the discovery of a whole range of new antibiotics. His expectations were soon fulfilled when, with the help of H. Boyd Woodruff, he isolated actinomycin and then streptothricin. Unfortunately, both these compounds proved far too toxic for use as antibiotics, although, as we shall see, actinomycin was later to be introduced as an antitumour drug.

The screening programme which yielded these compounds was essentially based on what has been described as 'a shotgun approach', that is, as many soils as possible were sampled and from these a wide range of actinomycetes were isolated and tested for their ability to produce antibiotics. The interesting isolates were then grown in large quantities of media and various chemical tricks were performed to extract the active ingredient. This was then exposed to animal toxicity and protection tests, and if it survived these then it was used in trials on humans. Waksman allocated a large proportion of this mundane screening work, as well as later studies on the physiology of any antibiotic producers, to his research students or research assistants. Herein lay the root of the problem which was to erupt with such force in the case of streptomycin, because while Waksman considered that he made the major intellectual contribution to the discovery of a given antibiotic, his students did not always agree with him. As far as some were concerned, it was their hard work and dedication which brought the new anti-biotics into being. This difference in outlook would eventually cause considerable misunderstanding, to the point of acrimony, between Waksman and one of his research assistants, Albert Schatz. It was Schatz who actually isolated one of the two streptomycin-producing strains of actinomycetes and laboured hard to extract and test the new antibiotic. On the completion of these studies, he wrote up the results in a thesis which was accepted by Rutgers in 1945, in part fulfilment of the degree of Doctor of Philosophy.

The discovery of streptomycin was first reported in a paper published in 1944 in *The Proceedings of the Society for Experimental Biology and Medicine*, under the title 'Streptomycin: a Substance Exhibiting Anti-biotic Activity Against Gram Positive and Gram Negative Bacteria.' The paper was published with Schatz's name first, followed by that of Elizabeth Bugie and finally Waksman. This order of names is in itself interesting, and was later to be the source of some argument. As a general rule, authors affix their names to scientific papers in order of those who contributed most of the laboratory work. However, it does not always follow that the first author made the major contribution to either the research or the resulting paper. Many PhD supervisors put their names last on a paper in order to advance the careers of their students. Waksman maintained that this was why Schatz's name headed the first streptomycin papers. It is relevant to note, however, that Waksman's publication list shows that on no previous occasion did he allow a student's name to appear first on a paper, so either he was being uncharacteristically generous to Schatz, or he recognized the unique contribution which the young man had made to the discovery of streptomycin.

The other interesting thing about this paper is that, while it mentions the fact that streptomycin can kill *Mycobacterium tuberculosis*, the cause of tuberculosis, it never dwells on the fact, nor is any prominence given to this crucial finding in the title of the paper. As a result, it has been argued that the Rutgers team at first failed to realize the full implication of what they had discovered. The title did, however, tell the reader that streptomycin, unlike penicillin, was capable of inhibiting both Gram-negative and Gram-positive bacteria, and as a result should have been useful in the treatment of a wide range of infections. However, the fact remains that there was little in this, the first

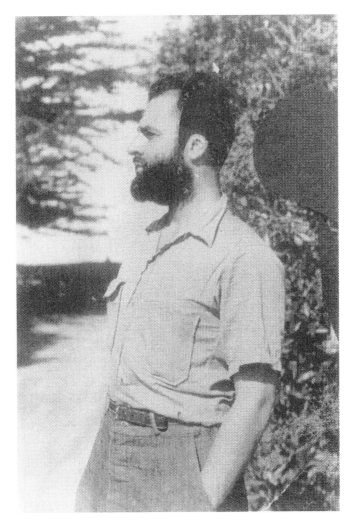

Plate 11 Albert Schatz, co-discoverer of streptomycin
(Pacific Grove California, 1949). (Courtesy of Professor
H. Seymour Hutner)

streptomycin paper, which would have given a tuberculosis sufferer immediate cause for rejoicing.

The next step would obviously be to extract and test the effectiveness of streptomycin on animals and then, provided all went well, on tuberculosis sufferers. As neither Waksman nor Schatz was medically qualified, nor experienced animal experimenters, this latter part of

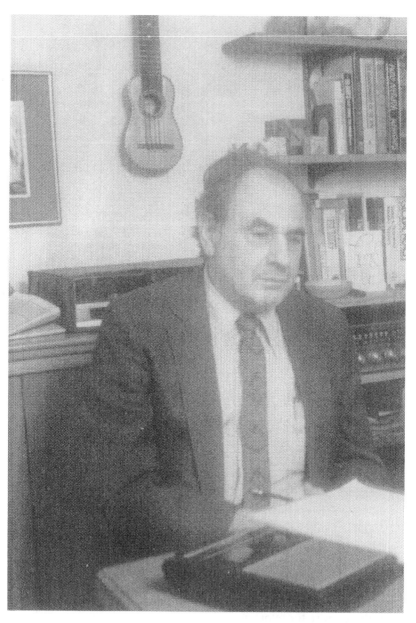

Plate 12 Albert Schatz as he is today. (Photograph by the author)

streptomycin's development would have to involve outside help. In the event, the task fell to two research physicians at the Mayo Clinic, in Rochester, Minnesota, William F. Feldman and H. Cornwin Hinshaw.

In 1894, at the age of 12, William H. Feldman had emigrated with his family to the States from Scotland. Although originally trained as a veterinary surgeon, he soon took a keen interest in human disease, and, after a two-year period as a pathologist at the Colorado State College, became a member of the full-time staff of the Division of Experimental Pathology at the Mayo Clinic. It was here that Feldman became particularly interested in comparative physiology, eventually using his expertise to write two major books on the subject, one being devoted to tuberculosis in birds, and the other to the subject of tumours in domesticated animals.

Hinshaw was also not originally trained in medicine, beginning his career in 1927 as an Assistant Professor of Zoology at the University of California at Berkeley. After obtaining his PhD, he spent the next three years as adjunct Professor of Parasitology and Bacteriology at the American University in Beirut, Lebanon. He then decided to seek medical qualifications, and in just two years of study, he obtained an MD from the University of Pennsylvania. In 1933, Hinshaw became a Fellow in Medicine at the Mayo Clinic, where he began to collaborate with Feldman on the experimental chemotherapy of tuberculosis.

The sulphonamides and penicillin had both failed miserably to influence the course of tuberculosis, and the opinion had become widespread that the tuberculosis bacillus, because of its protective, waxy coat, was somehow immune to the effects of antibiotics. Despite this pessimism, Feldman and Hinshaw continued to evaluate the anti-tubercular effects of a wide range of experimental drugs, beginning with the sulphone, promin, which incidentally was later to be used in combination with streptomycin to treat tuberculosis. Although this agent proved of no use in the treatment of tuberculosis, during its testing the Mayo Clinic scientists gained valuable insights into the best methods which could be used to evaluate the effectiveness of drugs against this disease.

News that the Rutgers team were looking for novel antibiotics prompted Feldman to write to Waksman, in July 1943, to enquire if one of the newly discovered compounds called clavicin was available to be tested against *Mycobacterium tuberculosis*. Waksman replied that clavicin was too toxic for use in humans but suggested that Feldman might like to visit Rutgers to discuss some alternatives.

Feldman met Waksman for the first time on 16 November 1943; it is not clear whether or not they discussed streptomycin. Schatz, in fact, gave the impression that the decision to test streptomycin against a virulent strain of M. *tuberculosis* was made after Feldman's visit, which implies that prior to this point, the Rutgers team were not particularly interested in concentrating upon finding a cure for tuberculosis.

In the months before Waksman next met Feldman, Schatz, aided by Elizabeth Bugie, was busy producing large quantities of streptomycin and discovering more about its properties. Streptomycin was found to be effective against *Shigella gallinarum*, the cause of fowl typhoid, *Salmonella scottmuleri*, a cause of food poisoning, and *Brucella abortus* and *Proteus vulgaris*, which respectively cause brucellosis and certain urinary tract infections. These preliminary trials were so promising that the pharmaceutical company, Merck, with whom Waksman had a long-standing agreement regarding patent rights on the Rutgers antibiotics, immediately set up a production plant at nearby Rahway, to provide the large quantities of purified streptomycin necessary for clinical trials. The demonstration by P. R. Heilman that streptomycin was effective in the treatment of tularemia, then an infection causing from 3 to 5 per cent fatality, added further impetus to this work, as did the realization that the new antibiotic could cure the unusually named disease 'Walking pneumonia', caused by *Klebsiella pneumonia*. These studies suggested that even if streptomycin failed to defeat tuberculosis, it would still play an important role in the treatment of a wide range of infectious diseases.

On 1 March 1944, Waksman once again contacted Feldman, this time to see if he was still interested in testing streptomycin against experimental tuberculosis. The Mayo Clinic team did not hesitate to confirm their interest, and, by April of that year, streptomycin had been tested on four guinea pigs which had been infected with the disease. The treatment continued until 20 June, when the samples ran out. However, even these limited tests proved promising, and on 10 July, Feldman and Hinshaw met with Waksman and a Merck representative to discuss how best to proceed. Then, from 18 July to the following September, further trials were conducted at the Mayo Clinic using new supplies of Merck purified streptomycin.

The guinea pig trials proved promising, but the crucial test was yet to come; would streptomycin cure tuberculosis or, for that matter , any other human infection?

STREPTOMYCIN'S FIRST CURES

The privilege of being the first person to be cured with streptomycin fell to a 2-year old boy who had been suffering from a heavy urinary infection, septicaemia and meningitis, causing him to become jaundiced and suffer from an enlarged liver and gall bladder. Streptomycin was given to the infant, and proved so successful that on 27 September 1944, Dr W. Richards of Columbia University, who had treated the child, wrote to Waksman expressing the excitement felt by all those at New York's Babies' Hospital who had taken part in the treatment.

However, another year was to elapse before streptomycin was used with success against tuberculosis. This treatment took place on 15 November 1945, when a 21-year old patient of Dr Karl Pfuetze was cured of pulmonary tuberculosis at the Mineral Springs Sanatorium in Canon Falls, Minnesota. By September 1946, Feldman and Hinshaw had treated some 34 cases of tuberculosis with streptomycin, but they remained cautious; perhaps it was impossible for them to believe that consumption really could be cured. On far too many occasions in the past, false hope had been raised in people who suffered from this disease. Now, however, there was real hope; at last there appeared to be an antibiotic which was not intimidated by the apparently impenetrable outer defences of *Mycobacterium tuberculosis*.

Like Florey before them, Feldman and Hinshaw received numerous letters pleading for samples of the meagre supplies of streptomycin then available, and as was the case with penicillin, shortages in supply of the new drug led to the development of a black market, with even samples of baking powder being peddled as streptomycin!

By 1944, the first large-scale clinical trial on the effectiveness of streptomycin against over 300 cases of tuberculosis was published by the Trudeau Society, soon to be followed by even more convincing trials, the first one carried out by the US Veterans Administration Hospital, and then an extensive British trial. These trials proved beyond all doubt that streptomycin was miraculously effective in the treatment of tuberculosis.

Then two storm clouds appeared on the horizon–streptomycin was not to be the troublefree cure for diseases like meningitis and tuberculosis for which hopes had been raised. However, before discussing these setbacks, it is worth dwelling for a while on the question of who deserves the credit for streptomycin's discovery and its introduction into medicine.

THE STREPTOMYCIN CONTROVERSY

The medical historian is presented with a major dilemma when allocating credit for the discovery of streptomycin. On the one hand, it is clear that it was Waksman who both began and led the research programme which led to the discovery of this antibiotic, while, on the other, it remains equally clear that it was Schatz who actually made the discovery and whose hard work led to it being produced in sufficiently large quantities to enable a proper evaluation of its medical properties. In addition we have to consider the involvement of Feldman and Hinshaw, whose research work at the Mayo Clinic led directly to streptomycin's introduction into medicine as an anti-tubercular drug.

Unfortunately, while due recognition fell to Feldman and Hinshaw, Waksman seemed loath to accept that Schatz was anything more than 'a pair of hands', a research assistant who worked under his close supervision and made no intellectual contribution whatsoever to the discovery.

Albert Schatz was born in Norwich, Connecticut on 2 February 1920. He first met Waksman in early 1941 while he was an under-graduate student at Rutgers. He showed considerable potential as a student and, on graduating, Waksman took him on as an assistant. However, while doing this work, which involved some screening work for antibiotics, he was drafted into the army and spent some time working in a medical laboratory. Here he became familiar with the methods used in handling pathogens, including the tubercle bacillus. Schatz was then invalided out of the army suffering from a recurrent back problem and he returned to Waksman's laboratory as a research student.

This change of status is important in relation to later events, because Schatz had changed from being one of Waksman's helpers to being a largely independent researcher. He had matured considerably while in the army and was quite capable of working on his own. Waksman assigned him the task of finding an antibiotic which was active against Gram-negative pathogens. Schatz agreed, because he was particularly keen to find a compound active against *Mycobacterium tuberculosis*. As he would be working with this and other pathogens, Waksman assigned him to a basement laboratory, where there would be little chance of the risk of accidental infection to others in the Agriculture Department. Waksman, it seems, was not too keen to be in a laboratory where the tubercle bacillus might be loose, and so rarely visited the laboratory, instead preferring that Schatz should come to his office to discuss the progress of his work. This fact on its own increased the independent nature of Schatz's work.

Prior to 1942, the relationship between Waksman and Schatz had been extremely friendly. After working with streptomycin and obtain-ing a Doctorate based on the work, Schatz left Rutgers to begin an independent scientific career and in 1949 found himself at the Hopkins

Marine Station, Pacific Grove in California. While working here, he frequently wrote to Waksman asking for advice on how best to further his career. Again the correspondence was extremely amiable, until 2 January 1949, when Waksman received a shock in the form of a letter from Schatz. Schatz began in a friendly enough manner: 'You have many times invited me to call upon you for advice that you may be in a position to render me, on either professional or personal problems.' Treading extremely carefully, Schatz went on to point out that by affixing his signature to every document which Waksman had sent him he had gradually been signing himself out of the credit and royalties rightly due to him from his part in the streptomycin discovery. Schatz then enquired about the financing of the Rutgers Research and Endowment Foundation which had been benefiting from the not inconsiderable monies now pouring in from the sale of streptomycin. In a series of questions, Schatz enquired about what had happened to these royalties, and in particular whether any individual was profiting from the discovery. This was an extremely pertinent question, because, before he left Rutgers, Schatz entered into a gentlemen's agreement with his supervisor that neither would profit from the discovery. Waksman had broken this agreement without informing Schatz and was now receiving considerable amounts in royalties from the Foundation. To be fair, much of the money he received was ploughed back into his research, or was used to fund trips to scientific conferences overseas. Nevertheless, he was clearly profiting from streptomycin, and to make matters worse he was forwarding small sums to Schatz but, instead of telling him where they were coming from, he appeared to act as a generous benefactor. The fact that Schatz was called upon to declare whether these monies were to be taxed as income or as gifts finally exposed Waksman's deceit.

Waksman's reply to his former research assistant's probing letter began: 'To say that I was amazed to read it is to put it quite mildly. I can assure you that it caused me considerable pain. I thought that this whole matter had been settled and buried.' Waksman then went on to point out that, as far as he was concerned, streptomycin was the product of a screening programme that had been set up before Schatz's arrival as an assistant at Rutgers. He admitted that Schatz had isolated one of the two streptomycin-producing strains of *Streptomyces griseus*, and also that he had assisted in the development of the methods used to isolate the crude material and test its antibacterial activity. He concluded, however, with the statement that he believed Schatz's contribution to comprise 'only a very small part of the picture in the development of streptomycin as a whole'. He then finished the letter with the following, somewhat ominous warning: 'I hope however, that you will reconsider this whole situation before it is too late. You have made a good beginning as a promising scientist. You have a great future and you cannot afford to ruin it.'

In a later letter, dated 8 February 1949, Waksman gave his account of the discovery in more detail. Again, his interpretation of the situation was quite straightforward: 'You were merely a cog in a great wheel in the study of antibiotics in this laboratory.' Waksman then listed ten important steps in the isolation of streptomycin, of which, he maintained, Schatz took part in only one, namely the isolation of one of the two streptomycin-producing strains. Waksman appears to have overlooked here two obvious points which indicate that Schatz played a more important role in the discovery than he credits him with in this letter. Firstly, as we have seen, Waksman allowed Schatz's name to go first on the early streptomycin papers. Perhaps more importantly, Schatz's name appeared on the patent application for streptomycin, and Waksman signed sworn affidavits to the fact that Schatz was indeed the co-discoverer. It is hard to imagine that Waksman would have been so generous to Schatz had the young man played only a minor role in the discovery.

The reader may wonder why I have not made reference to the apparently equally neglected role of Elizabeth Bugie, whose name also appears on the first streptomycin paper. The explanation is that, while Bugie contributed to the early work on streptomycin, she swore affidavits on the patent application to the effect that she played no part in the actual discovery of the antibiotic, and that Schatz and Waksman alone were co-discoverers.

The dispute between Schatz and Waksman eventually got completely out of hand. In the face of Waksman's intransigence, Schatz proceeded to issue a lawsuit against his former supervisor, demanding a share of the royalties for streptomycin and legal recognition as co-discoverer of the antibiotic. A long and drawn out civil court action followed in which Waksman's attorneys, in particular, pulled no punches.

One of the main points of contention at the hearing was the question of the origin of the streptomycin-producing strain which Schatz had isolated. The problem is compounded by the fact that there were two such strains. According to Waksman and his attorneys, the first was supplied by Fred Beaudette, the poultry pathologist at Rutgers. This strain was said to have been isolated from the throat of an infected chicken and then given to Waksman who then passed it onto Schatz. Schatz, on the other hand, maintained that this active strain was given to him by a fellow student called Doris Jones. She was one of Beaudette's students, and it was she who isolated the strain from the throat of a chicken. Doris Jones described what happened in the following words which were published in the *Rutgers University Douglas Bulletin* for 1977 (page 6): 'The strain of *Streptomyces griseus* [the streptomycin-producing strain] came from one of my culture plates. It was handed to Al Schatz through a basement window of the poultry pathology laboratory.' I was recently fortunate enough to discuss the origin of this strain with Doris Jones (now Doris Rolston), and she confirmed to me that she gave Schatz the streptomycin-producing strain and that it did not reach him via Beaudette and Waksman. A careful scrutiny of letters in the Waksman Archive at Rutgers also proves that Waksman, while initially stating that the strain came from Doris Jones, suddenly concluded, during the litigation proceedings, that it had reached Schatz from Beaudette, via himself as intermediary.

Waksman's attorneys suggested that Schatz's other streptomycin-producing strain, which he said had been isolated from soil, in fact arose as an accidental or perhaps even intentional transfer from what *they* called the Beaudette strain, i.e. that donated to Schatz by Doris Jones. They obviously did this in the hope that, if this could be proved, then Schatz's contribution to the discovery of streptomycin would be further diminished. In fact the two strains, although similar, were not identical, and the Schatz strain proved to be far more efficient in producing streptomycin than was the strain originating from the infected chicken. Not surprisingly, it was Schatz's strain which was used by Merck in the bulk production of streptomycin.

The lawsuit, brought by Schatz against Waksman, was a major source of embarrassment for Rutgers, and not surprisingly also generated something of a scandal in the scientific world. It is true to say that the scientific establishment closed ranks on Waksman's side and the few accounts of the streptomycin story which were not written by Waksman have tended to support Waksman and Rutgers, regarding Schatz as some ungrateful usurper of Waksman's good name. No mention of Schatz, the co-discoverer of streptomycin, is made by Waksman in the chapter of his autobiography, *My Life With the Microbes*, devoted to the discovery. The publicity department of Rutgers also ignored Schatz, instead portraying Waksman as the sole discoverer of streptomycin and as a humane benefactor, who had even refused to benefit financially from the discovery. However, there is no escaping the fact that Waksman reneged on the agreement he had with Schatz concerning streptomycin royalties. He also conveniently ignored the fact that both the patent documents and the contents of Schatz's thesis proved that Schatz was indeed entitled to be regarded as one of streptomycin's co-discoverers!

The streptomycin litigation continued throughout 1950, until finally the judge, doubtless confused by all the scientific jargon in use by both sides, decided to hear the case in his chambers. On 29 December 1950, the *New York Times* ran the headline 'Dr Schatz wins 3% of Royalty; named co-founder of Streptomycin'.

Eighty per cent of the royalties from streptomycin sales went to Rutgers, and much of this was used by Waksman to fund the Micro-biology Research Institute which bears his name. Waksman received 10 per cent, while the remaining 10 per cent was then distributed to all those students and scientists who played a role in the search for anti-biotics at Rutgers, including the laboratory dishwasher, a certain Mr Adams. Although Schatz received the largest share of this money, 3 per cent, he was against this settlement, because it made him appear as if he were but one of many people who had a hand in the discovery. The action brought by Schatz therefore not only enriched himself but brought relative wealth to other members of the Rutgers team, some of whom still criticize his actions! Also, unlike these people, Schatz had to pay his attorneys 40 per cent of the settlement which he received. One beneficial outcome of the streptomycin litigation was that it set a precedent so that students who were later to discover antibiotics at Rutgers automatically received royalty payments. Feldman, by the way, refused as a matter of principle to accept any of the royalties which were offered to him.

The settlement of the Schatz case did not, however, end the legal wrangles over streptomycin. In 1954, a certain Mary A. Marcus filed a complaint in the US District Court of New Jersey against both Waksman and Merck. The complaint maintained that Waksman had isolated streptomycin from some cultures which Marcus had given him in the 1920s, and since she was the inventor (sic) of streptomycin she was therefore entitled to compensation amounting to half a million dollars!

Fortunately, Waksman had no difficulty in disproving this wild allegation and in March 1956 the case was dismissed. This must obviously have been a distressing period for Waksman, especially as he received anonymous phone calls threatening the destruction of 'his reputation, and all that he loved' if he failed to settle the Marcus case. There must indeed have been many times during this period when Waksman regretted ever having heard of streptomycin!

THE NOBEL PRIZE FOR STREPTOMYCIN

As the 1945 Nobel Prize for Physiology or Medicine had been awarded for the discovery of penicillin, it was assumed by the general public that streptomycin would receive the same accolade. This was not the

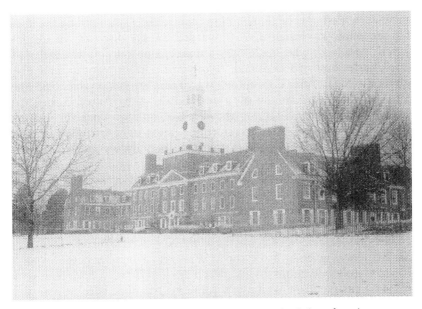

Plate 13 The Waksman Institute at Rutgers, built largely using streptomycin royalties. (Photograph by the author)

opinion generally held amongst the medical-scientific community, however, since many considered that the discovery of streptomycin was essentially an extension of the concept first realized by penicillin; in essence, they believed that it contributed nothing new to science. While this view undoubtedly has its merits, such rational thinking could not overcome the wave of emotion felt towards a drug that had apparently defeated tuberculosis. As a result, the 1952 Prize was awarded for the discovery of streptomycin, but only to Selman Waksman!

The reader may wonder why Albert Schatz, the legally defined co-discoverer of the new antibiotic, had been neglected, or, for that matter, why Feldman and Hinshaw did not travel to Stockholm with Waksman to receive the Prize. Unfortunately, since the deliberations of the Caroline Institute which awards this Prize are kept strictly confidential, we are unlikely ever to know the answers to these questions. However, by examining the limited number of documents on the subject which exist in the public domain, we can perhaps begin to understand why Waksman alone received the Nobel Prize for streptomycin.

The first point to understand about the committees which award the Nobel Prizes is that they are by no means infallible. Like all organizations, they make mistakes, and in the list of Prizes awarded over the years there have been some notable omissions as well as surprising inclusions. Perhaps the most famous controversy surrounding the Prize for medicine was when it was awarded for the discovery of insulin; J. J. R. Macleod, who made only a minor contribution, was included, but Charles Best was excluded. Another important point to remember about the Nobel Prize Committees is that they are answerable to no one, and, provided they follow the rules laid down by Alfred Nobel, can award the Prize to whomever they choose, and for whatever reasons. Put simply, they are under no direct obligation to be fair; they are after all administering a prize, and prizes do not always go to the most deserving! Having said this, the Nobel Prize has assumed an unequalled standing in the world of art and science, and it is because of its prominence that we expect that it will be allocated fairly and will accurately reflect the part played by all those involved in a major discovery, like that of streptomycin.

The presentation speech for the 1952 Nobel Prize for Physiology or Medicine was given by Professor A. Wallgren, a member of the Swedish Royal Caroline Institute. In his speech one can detect a certain amount of embarrassment on Wallgren's part that the prize is to be awarded only to Waksman. By including the names of Schatz, Feldman and Hinshaw, he appears to correct the injustice. More importantly, while the Prize was originally awarded to Waksman for 'his discovery of streptomycin, the first antibiotic effective against tuberculosis', Wallgren skilfully extends this, presenting Waksman with the award for what he describes as 'Your ingenious, systematic and successful studies of the soil microbes that have led to the discovery of streptomycin, the first antibiotic to remedy tuberculosis'. By this skilful interpretation of the reasons behind the offer of the award, Wallgren manages to diffuse any criticism about the award going only to Waksman. This is because, rather than awarding the Prize solely for streptomycin, he widens the parameters to include Waksman's work on soil microbiology as well as for the inception of the whole antibiotic screening programme. Had the Prize been given to Waksman from the outset for his magnificent contribution to soil microbiology and for his work on antibiotics, then no one could have questioned its allocation. Unfortunately, however, the 1952 Nobel Prize for Medicine was awarded to Waksman for *the discovery of streptomycin*, alone a fact which, since there was a co-discoverer, would inevitably lead to controversy and ill-feeling.

Not surprisingly, Schatz felt bitter about being denied a share of the Prize, and having successfully tasted blood over allocation of the streptomycin royalties, he was not about to let this omission go unchallenged. News of his omission from the Prize reached Schatz while he was Professor of Microbiology at the National Agricultural College,

Buck County, Pennsylvania. In response to the news, the Vice President of the College wrote to Professor Liljestrand, Secretary of the Nobel Prize Committee, on 29 October 1952 to make the following plea on Schatz's behalf: 'We are particularly gratified at this honour as the original discovery of streptomycin was jointly made by Dr Selman A. Waksman and Dr Albert Schatz, who is Professor of Microbiology at this College. We note, however, with some amazement that the award was made solely to Dr Waksman, one of the co-discoverers.' This statement was then followed by a detailed consideration of Schatz's case.

The reply from the Nobel Prize Committee was written by the President and Secretary, respectively, H. Bergstrand and G. Liljestrand. They stated that the information which had been forwarded had not been available to the Committees, and that when they had canvassed scientific opinion in the States and elsewhere no one had mentioned Schatz's name, let alone his involvement in the discovery. Such lame excuses obviously do not reflect well on the investigative qualities of the Nobel Prize Committees!

Schatz's pleading was doomed to failure; the Committees were never likely to alter their decision and the small agricultural college which was backing Schatz clearly did not have sufficient standing in the academic community to hope to correct the clear injustice. Undaunted as ever, Schatz wrote letters detailing his case to a number of eminent scientists and Nobel Prize winners including Fleming, Florey, Sabin and Krebs. Not surprisingly, none of these establishment figures decided to intercede on the young man's behalf. Perhaps Sabin gave the majority response to this pleading when he wrote to Waksman expressing his disgust that a postgraduate student should act in such an ungrateful and underhand way towards his former supervisor! The scientific establishment closed ranks and Schatz's name was lost almost for ever from the history of medicine. The consensus was that Waksman deserved the Nobel Prize for his long-term commitment to antibiotic research and discovery. This is a view, of course, which cannot be disputed, but it is important to keep on emphasizing that the Prize was given for the discovery of streptomycin *alone*. Where then was the legally and morally defined co-discoverer of the antibiotic?

In 1965, Schatz made one last attempt to put his side of the streptomycin story on record when he wrote an account of his work in the *Pakistan Dental Review*. This paper is a sad attempt by a young man to gain some measure of credit for his contribution to streptomycin. In it he recalls that he spent long hours working in the laboratory, often with little sleep. On one occasion he says that he was so exhausted that he fell into the snow outside the laboratory, and would have frozen to death had it not been for the efforts of a passing porter. The relationship between Waksman and Schatz portrayed in this article is a far cry from the warm letters which they wrote to one another before the streptomycin litigation destroyed their friendship for ever.

The streptomycin controversy can be viewed from a number of standpoints. There are those who say that Schatz was merely obeying Waksman's instructions and therefore made little in the way of an intellectual contribution to the discovery. If this were the case, then it would, as I have already said, appear strange that Schatz's name should figure so prominently, both on the streptomycin papers and on the patent application. Other people, perhaps reflecting on their own experience as a postgraduate, would recognize the high degree of commitment and skilful research which is generally required to obtain this qualification. There can be little doubt that Waksman's high-handed attitude to Schatz's contribution sowed the seeds of later acrimony. In retrospect, it is easy to suggest that Waksman should have been more forthcoming about the fact that he was receiving royalties on streptomycin, and that he should have taken a more charitable view of Schatz's contribution. It must be remembered, however, that Waksman belonged to the old school of European microbiologists, who regarded postgraduates as apprentices who were fortunate to be given an opportunity to work alongside a master in their chosen field.

Waksman gives his side of the streptomycin controversy in his autobiography. Nowhere in this account does he refer to Schatz by name, preferring instead to describe him as 'the former student'. Waksman explains the fact that he accepted monies for streptomycin, despite having agreed with Schatz not to, on the basis that they were offered for his efforts in helping Merck to develop the drug, rather than for the discovery itself. He also maintains that his motive in accepting these funds was to use them to advance his research, rather than to use them for personal gain. His explanation for the fact that Schatz's name was on the patent was as follows:

> It may be interesting to note that United States patent law requires that a patent application be executed by all co-inventors. It is sometimes difficult to distinguish between assistance and invention. In such cases, it is prudent that the patent application be executed by both the inventor and the assistant to avoid any possible legal defect, and that the assistant execute an assignment of his rights, if any, in the invention. Such was the case in the streptomycin patent to which was added the name of the former student.

These comments go some way to explaining why Waksman was totally unable to comprehend Schatz's point of view. To him, what might seem to us to be polite and justified probing about royalties, smacked of disloyalty and betrayal. Had Waksman taken the opposite stance then he could have appeared to history in a much better light. If this approach had been taken from the start, then there is little doubt that Schatz would have been more than happy to have taken a secondary role, standing in awe beside the man he had once so much respected and admired. The full tragedy of the contoversy can be summed up in Waksman's own words:

> As I look upon the year 1950, I consider it the darkest one in my whole life. Here I was at the height of my scientific career, acclaimed universally for having given to the world what promised to be a solution to the tuberculosis problem. Here I was about to be dragged into court and suffer indignities, at the instigation of one of my own students, whom I educated, to whom I had pointed a way in the field of science, and whom I believed capable of becoming one of the brilliant stars in a firmament of my group of students.

It is all the more tragic then that Waksman could not find the humility to offer Schatz his fair share of both the rewards and the glory that the co-discoverer of streptomycin rightly deserved.

STREPTOMYCIN: THE DREAM BEGINS TO FADE

The pharmaceutical firm of Merck, based in Rahway a few miles from Rutgers, soon began producing large quantities of streptomycin, first by surface culture and then deep fermentation methods. Unfortunately a number of unique problems soon began to emerge from this manufacturing process. The first was the appearance of what is termed an actinophage, that is a virus capable of infecting and destroying the streptomycin-producing culture. This setback at first threatened to completely halt the production of streptomycin, but, although it was eventually solved, it was to be followed by far more worrying clinical problems.

The first and most striking of these was the fact that while streptomycin was generally speaking non-toxic, the high doses necessary to cure tuberculosis caused unfortunate side effects. The symptoms included a ringing sound in the ears, vertigo, nausea, and nystagmus – a rapid involuntary movement of the eyeballs. In a few cases these symptoms were followed by a loss of balance and eventually total deafness. Tests were later to show that streptomycin and its derivative, dihydrostreptomycin, could attack the auditory and vestibular nerves which are responsible for both balance and hearing. Fortunately, these effects were largely dose-related and could be reduced by giving patients smaller doses of streptomycin. However, both Waksman and Schatz received pathetic letters from patients who, while cured of tuberculosis or meningitis, had tragically been made deaf by the drug. Often these letters demanded money to compensate for such damage. A particularly vitriolic example of the genre was sent to Schatz while he was fighting the streptomycin litigation. One can well imagine his grief, not only because the antibiotic which he had helped to discover was causing such distressing side effects, but also because, while he was receiving the blame, the fame, fortune and honour eluded him and went instead to Waksman!

Then yet another setback began to threaten streptomycin's status as a valuable, life-saving antibiotic. This problem surfaced when it was found that bacterial resistance to the drug was developing at an alarming rate. Some strains of bacteria actually seemed to require the compound in order to grow! Fortunately, two non-antibiotic drugs, isoniazid and PAS, came to streptomycin's rescue; when used in conjunction with the antibiotic they prevented the development of bacteria resistant to the antibiotic. The first signs of the development of such resistance came in early 1946, when Guy Youmans and E. H. Williston of Northwestern University reported that the amount of streptomycin required to inhibit the growth of some strains of the tubercle bacillus increased a thousandfold during therapy! The ability of para-aminosalicylic acid to inhibit *Mycobacterium tuberculosis* was first demonstrated in 1943 by the Swede, Jorgen Lehman. The new drug was used in clinical trials in the following year, and, while it proved to be capable of curing tuberculosis, it was by no means as effective as streptomycin. In the large doses required to achieve a cure, it also caused a number of unpleasant side-effects, such as nausea and diarrhoea. The obvious next step was to combine streptomycin and PAS, and to treat tuberculosis by what is termed 'combination therapy'. The search for new combinations, which, incidentally, involved Domagk of prontosil fame, led scientists in the USA and Germany almost simultaneously to isolate the hydrazide of isonicotinic acid. Later to be called isoniazid, this compound was shown to be dramatically successful when combined with streptomycin as a cure for tuberculosis.

Despite these setbacks, streptomycin continued to be manufactured and used in the treatment of a plethora of diseases including tuberculosis, leprosy, meningitis, empyema, pneumonia, gonorrhea, tularaemia and glanders. Its effect on tuberculosis is aptly summed up by these words from H. Cornwin Hinshaw, one of those who made its therapeutic use a reality: 'Since the discovery of streptomycin, tuberculosis death rates in the United States have been reduced to one-third of their former toll. No physician who cares for patients with tuberculosis will doubt that modern therapy deserves a large share of the credit for the survival of these many thousands of persons.'

Streptomycin was to prove to be the first in a long line of antibiotics derived from actinomycetes which have found a use in the treatment of tuberculosis, including viomycin, cycloserine, kanamycin, capreomycin and rifampin. When used in conjunction with isoniazid or PAS, streptomycin remains one of today's first-line drugs in the battle against tuberculosis. However, despite the advent of antibiotics capable of curing tuberculosis, the disease remains a major problem in the Third World, where some 50 to 100 million people are infected with the disease. Approximately three million people die each year from the disease, 80 per cent of the fatalities occurring in the Third World where antibiotics are presumably too expensive for general use. Clearly, then, the view that tuberculosis has been defeated world-wide is far from the truth.

Following the widespread use of streptomycin in medicine, Waksman toured the world as an honoured guest, and had many opportunities to see for himself the miraculous effect which the new antibiotic had on patients suffering from diseases like tuberculosis and meningitis. Wherever he travelled, he was given snapshots of children whose lives had been saved by streptomycin. These he kept in a series of scrapbooks which he called 'The Streptomycin Babies'. While in France, for example, he was introduced to two children, a boy called Michel and an 8-year old girl called Janet. Their doctor told him how they had been brought to the hospital six months previously, both in a coma suffering from tuberculosis, and how streptomycin treatment had saved their lives. Waksman poignantly described what happened when they met: 'The little girl curtsied. Both children grasped my hand, handed me their flowers and I patted their lovely heads. As I leaned over them I felt like crying. These two children had surely been saved by streptomycin.' There are many stories like these, lovingly presented in a collection of scrapbooks now held in the Waksman Archive at Rutgers. Their existence makes it even more tragic that the streptomycin story will forever by blighted by the quarrels between its co-discoverers, Schatz and Waksman.

Waksman died in 1973, at the age of 85, after having enjoyed a remarkably productive life. He authored or co-authored some 500 scientific papers and 28 books, and as well as being regarded as 'the father of the antibiotics' he is known as one of the doyens of the science of soil microbiology.

After leaving Waksman's laboratory and becoming embroiled in the streptomycin controversy, Albert Schatz continued a career in science, and was honoured for his role in the discovery of streptomycin by a few South American Universities. He was also awarded the Gold Medal of the Grand Prix Humanitaire de France by the French Government. In the mid-1970s he turned his attention from microbiology to the question of the desirability of fluorinating drinking-water supplies, arguing the case that such additions could be harmful to health, particularly amongst people suffering from malnutrition. At the time of writing Schatz is alive and well, living in Philadelphia. I recently had the privilege to meet him and his charming wife Vivian to discuss his role in the discovery of streptomycin. Schatz seemed to me to be a man with a remarkable intellect, who, despite the disappointments of his early scientific career, has made some fascinating and important contributions to subjects as diverse as microbiology, dental research, palaeontology and soil science. Schatz has also taken a keen professional interest in science education and most recently, like a number of other established, orthodox scientists, he has begun to take an interest in paranormal phenomena. By no means a rich man, it is clear that the streptomycin controversy had a profound impact on his life. He has been fortunate therefore to have been able to rely upon the continued support of his wife. Despite a renewal of interest in the streptomycin story the major role which he played in its discovery continues to be largely unknown.

9

Antibiotics Galore!

As we have seen, a considerable amount of interest was being shown in the subject of microbial antagonism during the late 1930s. However, this interest invariably related to the ecological role of the phenomenon, or to its possible application in the prevention of plant disease. One of the earliest such reports was published in the *Ohio Journal of Science*, by a US mycologist called Constantine Alexopoulos. Entitled *Studies on the Antibiosis Between Bacteria and Fungi*, this paper was published in 1938, so the work it described must have been underway at least during the preceding year. Although Alexopoulos was later to be one of the first to search for antifungal antibiotics, his name is more generally known from an excellent general mycological textbook called *Introductory Mycology* than as an antibiotic pioneer.

Soon after the appearance of penicillin as an antibiotic, research journals around the world began to fill with descriptions of new antibacterial compounds. Most of this early work was done by academic scientists, such as Waksman's group at Rutgers. It was not long, however, before the pharmaceutical companies set up their own screening programmes, and a range of new antibiotics would appear over the next decade or more earning this period the description of 'the golden age of antibiotics'.

Most people assumed that the supply of new, medically useful antibiotics would be almost unlimited. Ernst Chain certainly believed this to be true. He had arguments with Florey on a number of occasions because he felt that the lead which the Oxford team had already established with penicillin was being frittered away. His frustration on this point came across in the following words:

> I could not believe that we would not find other substances
> of equal, perhaps even greater versatility than penicillin. It
> was just too much to expect that Fleming had stumbled on
> the only antibiotic of use to man – the odds of this happening
> were astronomical. I saw a whole virgin field and we were
> the leaders and would remain so if we got enough money. I
> argued our position again and again with Florey and we had
> bitter fights.

As it happened, while Chain was correct in his belief that hundreds of
compounds capable of inhibiting pathogens would easily be found,
uncovering medically useful antibiotics would prove to be another
matter all together. Fleming's discovery, while not unique, turned out to
be very special indeed.

Except for the knowledge of how to isolate microorganisms and to
test their antibiotic-producing abilities, no particular expertise was
necessary to join this gold rush. This uncoordinated attempt at drug
discovery has often been described as a 'shotgun approach'. Hubert
Lechevalier, one of Waksman's students and co-discoverer of the
antibiotic neomycin, has even gone so far as to describe this type of
work as being 'silly simple'.

The golden age of antibiotics has often been portrayed as some kind
of heroic search for new life-saving drugs in the best altruistic tradition.
However, in reality, while such idealism did motivate some, the profit
motive became the overriding consideration. So much so that Albert
Schatz somewhat cynically referred to this period as the 'golden *dollar*
age of antibiotics'. It is noteworthy, however, that few antibiotics of any
significance have originated from behind the Iron Curtain, so the desire
for profits has clearly been a fundamental stimulus in the search for new
antibiotics.

An impressive roll call of antibiotics followed streptomycin onto the
medical scene, including chloramphenicol (1947), chlortetracycline
(1948), erythromycin (1952), vancomycin (1956), and gentamicin
(1963). In the last chapter we shall see that new antibiotics continue to
be discovered. They are also often put to more varied use than merely
killing pathogens. In 1972, for example, during a screening programme
directed towards the development of immunosuppressant compounds,
Jean Borel, working for Sandoz in Switzerland, discovered that cyclo-
sporin A (Sandimmun) possessed some interesting properties. The
compound was passed on to Professor Calne who showed that it could
prevent host cells from attacking transplanted cells, the commonest
cause of death after bone marrow transplantation.

Most new antibiotics originate from mass-screening programmes, and, as a result, there is little in the way of history associated with their discovery. However, there remain a few stories from the 'golden age of antibiotics', which form the subject of this chapter.

THE SEARCH FOR ANTIBIOTICS AT RUTGERS

We have already seen that numerous PhD students and research assistants worked with Selman Waksman during the early 1940s in the screening of soil actinomycetes, leading to the discovery of a number of antibiotics, including the most important of all – streptomycin. In 1937, Waksman, together with Jackson W. Foster, published the second of the three papers which he co-authored in that year on the subject of microbial antagonism in which the following words are included:

> Different soil organisms found amongst the fungi, ascomycetes, and bacteria are capable of producing, when grown on synthetic media, substances which are antagonistic to the growth of other soil organisms. A detailed study has been made of the antagonistic effect of one species of actinomycetes upon a variety of fungi, bacteria, and other actinomycetes. The inhibiting effect produced by this organism was shown not to be due to exhaustion of nutrients or to unfavourable changes in reaction, but was found to be specific in nature. The maximum production of the antagonistic substance took place in the culture of the actinomycetes 7 to 18 days old. The substance was then gradually destroyed. Aeration and heat brought about rapid destruction of the substance.

From this statement, it is clear that Waksman had begun to understand the true nature of antibiotics. While he made no mention of the possibility of applying these observations to medicine, it is apparent that, once this possibility had been demonstrated by the work of Florey and Chain on penicillin, Waksman was ideally placed to begin his search of actinomycetes with the ability to produce medically useful antibiotics.

The first compound of interest to result from this work was actinomycin, which was isolated in 1940 from *Actinomyces antibioticus* by Waksman and one of his research assistants, H. Boyd Woodruff. In collaboration with Max Tishler, a chemist at Merck, actinomycin was crystallized and found to contain two compounds, one a red substance, actinomycin A, which was unfortunately too toxic to be used in other antibiotic-producing strains of actinomycetes. In August 1942, Waksman, working with E. S. Horning and E. L. Spencer, announced the isolation of two further antibiotic substances: fumigacin and clavacin. Both were produced by species of fungi belonging to the genus *Aspergillus*: the former by *A. fumigatus*, while clavacin was produced by *A. clavatus*. Fumigacin was active against Gram-positive bacteria and was mildly toxic; therefore, although its activity was similar to penicillin, it was abandoned because it was more dangerous to use. Clavicin had a broad spectrum of activity, being effective against both Gram-negative and Gram-positive bacteria. Unfortunately its toxicity was almost as great as that of actinomycin and therefore it could not be considered for use by intravenous injection.

In view of the fact that penicillin had become well established in the treatment of infections caused by Gram-positive bacteria, Waksman decided to turn his attention to the isolation of antibiotics which would inhibit Gram-negative pathogens. This approach realized streptothricin in 1942, a compound which proved to be capable of inhibiting pathogenic bacteria and even fungi in experimental animals. Unfortunately, however, just at the point when it might have been produced commercially, streptothricin was shown to have a delayed toxic effect on animals.

Surprising as it may now appear, Waksman's work did not attract US Government funding. The reply to an application to the Committee on Medical Research of the National Defense Research Council was apparently typical of the responses which he received to grant requests to extend his highly promising work: 'What you propose to do is purely theoretical; it can wait until the war is over. If you want to work on penicillin, you can have all the funds you require.' Waksman's work was not even considered important enough to exempt male students from the draft, and as a result, men like Schatz were drafted into the army, which helps to explain the preponderance of women in Waksman's laboratory at that time. Nevertheless Waksman did receive funds to finance his search for antibiotics from actinomycetes. The money, some $9,600 over six years, was generously provided by a private foundation called the Commonwealth Fund.

Waksman made up for the lack of government funding by forging close links with Merck. The company provided assistance with the chemical purification of the antibiotics isolated in Waksman's laboratory, as well as any help needed with bacteriological and pharmacological studies. In return, Merck was given first refusal on any promising compounds which might result.

This agreement with Merck was, as we have seen, to produce mutual financial rewards, particularly as a result of sales of streptomycin. The continued search for antibiotics in Waksman's laboratory increasingly produced dividends throughout the forties and fifties. Some of the compounds unearthed, like grisein, which was discovered by Reynolds and Schatz, were to find no practical use in medicine. Others, like neomycin, discovered by another of Waksman's research assistants, Hubert Lechevalier, proved more promising. However, after initial hopes that neomycin might be used in conjunction with streptomycin in the treatment of tuberculosis, it was relegated to a relatively minor role in the treatment of topical and oral bacterial infections. This antibiotic, however, is quite extensively used in the treatment of diarrhoea in infants and also to eliminate the normal and pathogenic flora of the intestine prior to surgery.

With the discovery of neomycin there surfaced a problem which is still very apparent today, relating to the discovery of similar compounds by researchers in various parts of the world who, in believing that they are working with a novel compound, give it a different name and thereby cause considerable confusion. Thus neomycin was isolated in Japan, France and the Soviet Union and given names such as colimycin, framycetin and meserin. Fortunately, and perhaps surprisingly, these independent discoveries of neomycin did not lead to long and costly legal arguments about patent rights.

Waksman often liked to give the impression that the discovery of each new antibiotic required the screening of thousands of soil isolates, making it indeed an heroic task. However, in a recent letter to Waksman's son Byron, Hubert Lechevalier put the screening programme into context as follows:

> You were right to say that your father liked to tell the 10, 000 or was it 100, 000 cultures story? In practice each student screened only a few hundred cultures. You have to remember that at that time all antibiotics were new and that finding an antibiotic-producing culture was not a rare event. I have never seen notebooks here presenting evidence that thousands and thousands of cultures had been screened. The story tells more about your father as a story teller than it gives a true picture of the screening programme in the Department. In my own case, the screening of 172 cultures yielded both the neomycin and the candicidin-producing strains.

The search for antibiotics at Rutgers continued with the establishment of the Waksman Institute, although Waksman became less directly involved in the work as the years slipped by. Recent compounds to emerge from this illustrious 'stable' include candihexin and hydro-heptin. In general, however, as we shall see later, the large-scale screening programmes have left the domain of the academic research department so that most of the recently introduced antibiotics originate from mass-screening programmes initiated by the world's major chemical-pharmaceutical companies. The part played by Waksman and his various associates in the antibiotic story is perhaps best summed up by these words of Ernst Chain:

> Dr Waksman's interest in antibiotics stems directly from his own subject, soil microbiology, and he was well acquainted with the phenomenon of microbial antagonism. I have no doubt that the intensive screening effort on soil organisms in the early and middle forties was speeded up by the publication of our papers on the curative properties of penicillin. However, I would like to point out that Dr Waksman would have been successful sooner or later in the discovery of the chemotherapeutically active antibiotics. Even if we had done no work on penicillin, and even if Fleming had not published his paper in 1929, Waksman's screening programme would have led sooner or later to the discovery of all useful antibiotics including penicillin. In conclusion, the role of Dr Waksman in the development of the field of antibiotics is really of primary importance and the world has recognized this by the numerous high awards he has received including the Nobel Prize which he richly deserved.

The Fungus Fighters

Most of the killer diseases from which mankind suffers are caused either by bacteria or viruses. Fungi, on the other hand are regarded as generally benign organisms which rarely act as pathogens. However, as we saw earlier, some species, including a number of yeasts, do cause infections, although many of these diseases prove to be troublesome rather than fatal. Nevertheless, the annual cost of treating this type of infection in the US alone reaches some 75 million dollars! Troublesome but hardly life-threatening diseases caused by fungi include athlete's foot and ringworm (referred to as dermatoses or dermatophytoses), while more worrying diseases include vaginal thrush, which is an infection of the mucous membranes caused by the yeast *Candida albicans*.

In some countries fungi are far more important as pathogens and produce what are referred to as 'deep mycoses'. These include potentially fatal infections such as histoplasmosis, a cause of severe damage to the liver and central nervous system. Life-threatening fungal infections are becoming more common, particularly amongst patients whose immune systems have been artificially suppressed, for example, prior to receiving organ transplants, or where immunity has been naturally suppressed by diseases like AIDS. Other patients who are likely to be immunosuppressed include those suffering from leukaemia, lymphoma, cancer victims receiving chemotherapy, diabetics, and patients receiving large doses of steroids. Even broad-spectrum antibiotics can increase a patient's susceptibility to fungal infections. In these cases fungi, which are generally considered to be nonpathogenic, take advantage of the host's reduced immunity to cause infections. For example, in one US hospital, a staggering 20 per cent of deaths in patients with acute leukaemia were caused by fungi, while a third of the deaths in a kidney transplant centre resulted from fungal infections! In nearly all cases, deep mycoses result when airborne spores are breathed into the lungs. Even ubiquitous fungi such as species of *Fusarium* and *Aspergillus*, more commonly known as decomposer organisms or plant pathogens, can fatally infect such compromised patients. In these people such fungi find a particularly hospitable environment for growth. Most of us can inhale the spores of the fungi causing these infections without apparent ill effect, or at worst suffering only minor respiratory problems. In some people, however, signs of distress may soon appear, or else the infection may lie dormant, and the symptoms then appear some years later. Unfortunately, many of these infections can be incorrectly diagnosed by doctors who are often unfamiliar with the symptoms they cause. This problem is compounded by the fact that many of the symptoms of these infections mimic those of a number of bacterial diseases, such as pneumonia and tuberculosis. However, deep mycoses are fortunately generally restricted to defined geographical areas, where the symptoms they produce are well known and can be adequately diagnosed and rapidly treated.

A wide range of opportunistic infections caused by fungi are seen in AIDS patients, and in fact the occurrence of these infections is frequently used as a criterion for defining the presence of the syndrome. Pneumonia, encephalitis and meningitis due to fungi such as *Aspergillus*, *Candida Cryptococcus*, or pathogenic *Zygomycetes* are all frequently diagnosed amongst AIDS sufferers. The presence of oesophageal candidiosis and cryptococcosis of the central nervous system are particularly valuable indicators of AIDS. Skin infections caused by fungi are also common, including severe and prolonged foot infections and a form of nail invasion where the fungus attacks from the nail base rather than, as is usual, from the outer or side edges. A common occurrence amongst AIDS patients are viral mouth ulcers, caused by the *Herpes simplex* virus, which are often super-infected with *Candida albicans*. *Candida* is a commensal yeast which also infects the gut of these patients, from where it invades the vital organs, including the brain. Without doubt, however, the mycosis found in AIDS patients which is the most time-consuming in terms of treatment is cryptococcosis. This deep, severe infection was until 25 years ago invariably fatal. From 1978 to 1983 cryptococcosis was found in some 6 to 13 people in the UK; at that time all were non-AIDS sufferers. In 1988, however, 28 cases were reported, of which 22 were AIDS related. Doctors who treat AIDS patients are increasingly coming across rare and what might even be called 'exotic' fungal infections. For example, an AIDS patient who spent some time in South China recently presented doctors in England with a deep mycosis caused by *Penicillium marneffei*, which was previously known only as a pathogen of the Vietnamese bamboo rat! Fortunately, as we shall see later, many of these fungal infections which inflict themselves upon AIDS sufferers are treatable, at least in the short term, with antibiotics.

One of the first attempts to use microorganisms to cure a fungal infection in humans did not involve the isolation and use of an antibiotic in the strict sense, but rather a living bacterial culture. As a result, this early attempt at a cure was similar to the recent use of living cultures of lactobacilli to treat mucosal yeast infections, a subject which we will look at in more detail later in this section. The first systematic attempt to cure a fungal infection using bacteria came in 1927 when Stanley Chambers and Fred Weidman, of the Department of Dermatology at the University of Pennsylvania, cured severe cases of ringworm of the toes using cultures of *Bacillus subtilis*. This pioneering work was done the year before Fleming's discovery of penicillin, and once again demonstrates how some workers clearly understood the potential use of microbial antagonism in the treatment of infections. The clinical trials conducted by Chambers and Weidman were apparently successful in 50 per cent of cases, causing them to conclude their paper with the following words: 'The principle underlying this experiment, i.e., the action of associated antagonistic micro-organisms, met with sufficient success to encourage its application to other dermatoses in which the causative micro-organism is known and is cultivable.' Some years later, in the early 1950s, it was found that a number of bacteria, including *B. subtilis*, produce antifungal polypeptides, thereby providing a rationale for the apparent effectiveness of Chambers and Weidman's methods. However, nothing seems to have become of this approach to the therapy of fungal infections, the effective treatment of which had to await the antibiotic era.

Albert Schatz, the co-discoverer of streptomycin, was amongst the first to try and find an antibiotic effective against fungi. After leaving Waksman's laboratory at Rutgers, he moved on to the Division of Laboratories and Research at Albany, New York. Here he worked with Elizabeth Hazen on a screening programme aimed at isolating actinomycetes with the ability to produce antifungal agents.

Elizabeth Lee Hazen was born on 24 August, 1885, in a small farming village called Rich in Mississippi. In 1905, she enrolled at the Mississippi Industrial Institute and College at Columbus, which had been founded in 1884, as the first state-supported college for women in the USA. After a short period as a teacher, she obtained an MA and later a PhD at Columbia University in New York.

In 1948, Hazen and Schatz published a paper describing how they obtained a number of active isolates, although they were unable to obtain compounds which were both effective antifungal agents and at the same time non-toxic. Schatz then moved onto more academically demanding scientific research, while Hazen continued to search for antifungal antibiotics. Following the departure of Schatz she realized that in order to be successful she would need to form a partnership with a chemist, who could isolate any active ingredients which her actinomycetes produced. As a result Hazen began collaborating with a chemist called Rachel Brown, and so began one of those 'double acts' which have proved so productive in science.

Rachel Brown was 13 years Elizabeth Hazen's junior. Born in Springfield, Massachusetts, she came from a relatively well-to-do background. Like her colleague, she began her working life as a schoolteacher before obtaining a first degree and then PhD in chemistry from the University of Chicago.

Together, Hazen and Brown would discover nystatin, the first truly successful antifungal antibiotic. Perhaps the use of the word 'together' here is somewhat inappropriate, as the two scientists worked in different laboratories, separated by some 150 miles!

After some preliminary studies, Hazen and Brown decided to redouble their efforts to isolate soil actinomycetes. One culture had, in fact, been left for further study by Albert Schatz, but, as was becoming the norm, while this strain produced an antibiotic it proved too toxic for clinical use. So Hazen and Brown next turned their attention to an actinomycete designated strain 48240. This organism yielded two antibiotic compounds, one which was poorly soluble in water – a fact which appeared to limit its medical use – while the other compound turned out to be an already established antibiotic.

Despite its apparent drawbacks, Hazen and Brown nevertheless concentrated on the first compound, giving it the name fungicidin. The strain of actinomycete which yielded this antibiotic was named *Streptomyces noursei* in honour of Hazen's friend Walter B. Nourse, from whose farm the soil sample containing the isolate had originally been obtained. The word fungicidin, it turned out, had been used previously to describe another antibiotic, so Hazen and Brown renamed their new antifungal compound nystatin, a word which originated as a corruption of 'New York State', in which it had been extracted.

The responsibility for handling the patenting and licensing of nystatin to an experienced pharmaceutical company was handed over to a charitable foundation for the advancement of science called the Research Foundation. Hazen and Brown, for their part, decided that most of the royalties they received on the antibiotic should be ploughed back into science to fund research, particularly in the then neglected area of medical mycology. In March 1951, the Research Foundation entered into a manufacturing agreement with the pharmaceutical company E. R. Squibb, who began producing fungicidin, as it was then still called, at their plant in New Brunswick, New Jersey. Deep fermentation techniques were employed, at first using 800 gallon tanks, which were then followed by tanks containing some 18,000 gallons of fermentation broth. The US patent on fungicidin was held up because initially no evidence of 'utility' had as yet been provided. This requirement could only be met following extensive clinical trials on humans. Eventually, patents were granted and in August 1954, Squibb began marketing the new antibiotic under the trade name 'Mycostatin'. In September of that year, Mycostatin was marketed in tablet form and recommended for use in the treatment of moniliasis and candidiasis. Shortly after the introduction of Mycostatin, Squibb marketed a mixture of this antibiotic and the antibacterial agent tetracycline. Although banned in the US because of lack of proof of efficacy, these antibacterial-antifungal mixtures were extensively used in other parts of the world. A total of over 13 million dollars was paid in royalties for nystatin over the period 1955 to 1976, of which nearly seven million went into the Brown-Hazen Fund, which was for many years the largest single source of non-federal funding in the US for research and training in medical mycology.

Although both Hazen and Brown received numerous awards, they were denied the Nobel Prize for their discovery, a fact which doubtless reflects the low priority given by the medical profession to fungal infections. Elizabeth Hazen died in 1975, at the age of 89, while Rachel Brown survived her, dying at the age of 81 in 1980.

Griseofulvin is another antifungal antibiotic, one which had an unusual origin. In 1939, Raistrick and Simonart, working at Oxford

University, described a metabolite isolated from the fungus *Penicillium griseofulvum*. Although they worked on the chemistry of this metabolite, they did not look at its biological activity. Then in 1946, Brian, Curtis and Hemming independently isolated a substance from *Penicillium janczewskii* which caused the filamentous structures, hyphae, of another fungus, *Botrytis allii*, to grow in a stunted and curled fashion. They named this substance 'curling factor'. The original strain of the *Penicillium* producing this factor was isolated from soils of a newly planted conifer forest on Wareham Heath in Dorset. These soils were interesting because they appeared somehow to prevent the development of certain mycorrhizae, fungi which live on the root surface and which promote plant growth. Further studies were to show that the Oxford metabolite and the 'curling factor' were one and the same compound. This was isolated by Grove and McGowan at ICI and given the name griseofulvin. Griseofulvin was used against fungal infections in plants for quite some time, but it was not until 1958 that its effectiveness in treating animals was realized, when J. C. Gentles, a mycologist in the bacteriology department at Anderson's College Medical School in Glasgow, reported its successful use in inhibiting pathogenic fungi in artificially infected guinea pigs. Griseofulvin can be administered orally, but is particularly extensively used in the treatment of superficial fungal infections of the skin.

Nystatin and griseofulvin continue to be widely used, especially in the treatment of skin infections and those caused by mucosal yeasts. To some extent, however, these older generation of antifungal compounds have been superseded by newer antibiotics such as amphotericin (Fungizone). This antibiotic is produced by yet another actinomycete, *Streptomyces nodosus*, which was originally from the Orinoco River region of Venezuela. While amphotericin can be used to treat systemic infections, particularly those which threaten the lives of patients with compromized immune systems, it unfortunately also produces serious side effects, such as fever, nausea and anorexia, and so is by no means the ideal antifungal antibiotic. The search for that continues.

THE BROAD-SPECTRUM ANTIBIOTICS

As their name suggests, these compounds inhibit a wide range of both Gram-positive and Gram-negative bacteria, and as a result, can be used to treat a wide range of infections. The story of the first of these compounds begins with a moonlit walk in 1943 on Gibson Island in Chesapeake Bay. The strollers, Paul R. Burkholder and Oliver Kamm, were attending a conference held by the American Chemical Society.

Burkholder was a Yale University microbiologist, while Kamm was director of the giant pharmaceutical firm, Parke Davis. Kamm had already been involved in the industrial development of some of the early antibiotics and was now looking at ways by which his company could become more extensively involved in the antibiotic business. On that moonlit stroll, he suggested to Burkholder that it might be worthwhile looking for antibiotics which had a very broad spectrum of activity.

Burkholder took something of a novel approach to the task of isolating such a compound. Instead of merely testing soil samples from his immediate neighbourhood, he asked his friends and colleagues scattered all over the world to fill a container with some of their local soil. As a result, he was able to isolate around 7,000 actinomycetes, of which nearly 2,000 inhibited *Staphylococcus aureus* to a greater or lesser extent. From these, however, he was eventually to produce only four isolates which showed any real promise as producers of medically useful antibiotics. One of these isolates, named *Streptomyces venezuelae* due to its South American origins, yielded an antibiotic which was at first given the trade name of Chloromycetin, but was later to become better known as chloramphenicol.

Chloromycetin, which was the first antibiotic to be fully synthesized, had already demonstrated its worth by 1947, when a typhus epidemic broke out along the Peru–Bolivia border. For one victim of the epidemic, a certain Gregario Zalles, treatment could not have come at a more opportune moment, as arrangements for his funeral were already in hand!

Unfortunately, the use of chloramphenicol was to be dramatically curtailed when it was discovered that it caused a form of aplastic anaemia. Not surprisingly, the profits of Parke Davis, who had sole manufacturing rights to this antibiotic, experienced an equally dramatic collapse.

While Parke Davis were assessing the value of chloramphenicol, their rivals, Lederle Laboratories, were looking for new anti-tuberculosis drugs to replace streptomycin. This research programme was headed by Benjamin M. Duggar, a 72-year old former Professor of Botany at the University of Wisconsin.

Duggar had been screening soils from all over the world, hoping to isolate new antibiotic-producing actinomycetes. In all, he had screened some 7,000 isolates before finding an unusual golden-coloured culture, which he named *Streptomyces aureofaciens*. Labelled strain number A377, this organism, isolated from a soil sample from Columbus, Missouri, yielded an antibiotic which was released into the world as aureomycin, but became better known as chlortetracycline. This compound proved to be a true broad-spectrum antibiotic, and soon became one of the most frequently prescribed drugs in medicine.

Both chloramphenicol and the tetracyclines proved particularly effective in the treatment of an infection called Rocky Mountain Spotted Fever. This disease, which is known throughout the USA under a variety of names such as tick fever, or bull fever, is not restricted to the Rocky Mountain region, but occurs in all but one of the States of the Union. It is an acute infection caused by a type of bacterium called a rickettsia, the most well-known example of which causes typhus. These organisms are very difficult to culture in the laboratory and can only be studied when growing in chicken eggs or in infected animals. Rocky Mountain Spotted Fever is transmitted to humans by a tick, and as a result, the disease is particularly common amongst farmers, forest rangers and campers. It is a seasonal disease, which in the USA occurs most frequently during June. The symptoms of Rocky Mountain Spotted Fever take a characteristic course, beginning a few days after a tick bite with a high fever, severe prostration, headache, deep soreness of the bones and muscles and a phobia towards light. The body temperature then increases to 104°F, and a rash develops on the hands and feet. Mental confusion and delirium are common, leading to death. By 1944, Rocky Mountain Spotted Fever was being successfully treated, first by chloramphenicol and then, in 1948, using aureomycin; finally both the incidence and severity of this distressing disease were reduced by the appearance of a specific vaccine.

By 1949, Pfizer had discovered what they thought was a new broad-spectrum antibiotic, which they named terramycin. However, it was soon shown to be identical to aureomycin. Nevertheless, patent rights battles over the tetracyclines continued for some time, and were amongst the most bitter ever fought. They destroyed once and for all any idea that the search for antibiotics was based on idealism rather than the search for multi-million dollar profits!

THE CEPHALOSPORINS: ANTIBIOTICS FROM A SEWAGE MICROORGANISM

As we have already seen, by far the majority of microorganisms known to produce important antibiotics were originally isolated from soils, and turned out to be actinomycetes. Penicillin provides an obvious exception to this rule, being produced by a fungus isolated as an airborne contaminant. A similar exception is provided by cephalosporin, an antibiotic produced by a fungus with a somewhat unusual origin. The cephalosporins have become the most widely used group of antibiotics. They are closely related to the penicillins, and like these have a β lactam ring at their active site which inhibits bacterial cell wall synthesis.

In 1945, Giuseppe Brotzu, Professor of Bacteriology at Cagliari University on the Island of Sardinia, took a more logical approach to the isolation of antibiotic producers than the usual 'shotgun method'. He concluded that sewage effluent might be a rich source of microorganisms antagonistic to the typhoid bacillus, and so began isolating organisms from a local sewage outfall which discharged into the sea. His labours resulted in the isolation of an antibiotic-producing strain of a fungus called *Cephalosporium acremonium*, from which the antibiotic obtained its name – cephalosporin.

Brotzu described his work in a rather obscure, privately published pamphlet called the *Works of the Institute of Hygiene of Cagliari*, only a single issue of which ever seems to have been published. It appears that, in the troubled circumstances in Italy following the Second World War, Brotzu had difficulty finding a journal which would publish his work. His response was quite novel; he merely invented his own! Brotzu describes producing a crude extract prepared by adding alcohol to the culture filtrate. This had a wide antibacterial spectrum, and was successfully used by Brotzu to treat boils and abscesses. The concentrated extract was even injected into patients suffering from typhoid, paratyphoid and brucellosis, apparently with good results.

Fortunately, Brotzu sent a copy of this pamphlet to Dr Blyth Brooke, a British public health officer who was working on the island. A sample of the mould was forwarded to Florey in Oxford, who then passed it on to Heatley for further evaluation. However, at that moment, Heatley was involved in some work on another antibiotic, called micrococcin, which incidentally was also isolated from a sewage organism. Brotzu's antibiotic was therefore worked on by E. P. Abraham, Kathleen Crawford and H. S. Burton working in collaboration with the MRC Antibiotics Research Station at Clevendon. The first stage of this research yielded a product which was named cephalosporin P, because of its activity against Gram-positive bacteria. Both chemically and in terms of its antibiotic spectrum this compound resembled helvolic acid. Clinical trials on cephalosporin P were undertaken by Glaxo, but they came to nothing. Interestingly, this antibiotic has a similar structure to fusidic acid which was recently evaluated as a possible AIDS cure, and about which we will hear more later.

At this point, Burton left, and his place was taken by Guy Newton. The new team discovered that there was a second antibiotic in the culture medium, which they named cephalosporin N, a compound which turned out to be closely related to penicillin. The name of this antibiotic was later changed to penicillin N and it found a use in the treatment of typhoid, replacing the more toxic chloramphenicol for this purpose. It turned out that cephalosporin N was the major antibiotic component which had first attracted Brotzu's attention.

The team persevered with their studies and eventually detected traces of a third antibiotic in the culture medium produced by Brotzu's isolate. Called cephalosporin C, this compound, while having a relatively low antibiotic activity, had the ability to withstand the action of the enzyme penicillinase. Then, in 1957, workers at the Clevendon Research Station isolated a high cephalosporin C-yielding mutant of the mould, which justified industrial production of the new penicillinase-resistant antibiotic. Just at that time, however, a collaboration between Chain and Beecham's bore fruit with the appearance of methicillin, the first of the semi-synthetic penicillins. Beside methicillin, cephalosporin P looked like a distinct commercial failure. Then, fortunately, it was realized that its side chain could be removed and replaced by others which led to an enhancement of its antibacterial activity. The chemical problems involved in achieving these replacements proved considerable however, and it was not until the 1960s that the full potential of the cephalosporins was realized.

By 1978, annual sales of the cephalosporins exceeded even those of the semi-synthetic penicillins. On this occasion, the British, including Florey and members of the Oxford team, were to benefit financially from the introduction into medicine of a new antibiotic. Sadly, Guy Newton was not to enjoy the fruits of his labours as he died at the early age of 49, on New Year's Day, 1969.

The lowly fungus isolated from a sewage outfall therefore turned out to have a bigger impact on the history of medicine than anyone could at first have imagined.

PATULIN: A FAILURE OF THE GOLDEN AGE OF ANTIBIOTICS

Although numerous attempts were made to isolate an antiviral antibiotic during the early years of the antibiotic era, it soon became apparent that there would be no easy panacea against this type of infection. One viral infection that most people assumed would soon fall a victim of the antibiotics was the common cold. If an antibiotic could be found capable of curing the infamous killer diseases like tuberculosis and pneumonia, then surely, it was argued, a trivial infection like the common cold should present few problems for medical science.

The miseries associated with colds need no elaboration here, especially for British readers. When news came in 1943 that an antibiotic had been found that could relieve cold symptoms, it met with considerable excitement. If effective, such a cure would prove a tremendous boon to the war effort.

The apparent breakthrough was reported in the medical journal *Lancet* by a team of scientists led by Harold Raistrick. Raistrick, it will be remembered, had been involved in early attempts to purify penicillin. Now he was claiming that his group had found an antibiotic called patulin, which could cure the common cold.

The realization that this compound was apparently effective against colds came by accident, when, soon after it was isolated, a sample was sent to a certain Dr W. E. Gye. At the time that he received the sample, Gye was suffering from a bad head cold and so decided to see if the new antibiotic might relieve some of his symptoms. He began this self-treatment by douching his nasal passages with a concentrated solution of patulin. The treatment caused him some pain, but he claimed that within an hour some of his symptoms had been noticeably reduced, and after another couple of treatments he was able to enjoy the first good night's sleep for some time. The following morning, he was feeling fit enough to return to work where he excitedly extolled the virtues of his new treatment. When two of Gye's friends reported similar curative effects of patulin treatment on their cold symptoms, it was decided to evaluate the claims by setting up a full-scale clinical trial. Organized by W. A. Hopkins, Surgeon Commander of the Royal Navy, this trial was carried out during the first four months of 1943, at a naval establishment 'somewhere in the south east of England'. In some cases, patulin was sprayed up the noses of the naval 'volunteers' while others sniffed it as a dry powder. The results of this trial proved very encouraging, with 54 per cent of the treated cases claiming relief from cold symptoms within 48 hours, compared with less than 10 per cent success amongst the control group. The data obtained from this trial were then statistically analyzed and the results seemed to prove beyond doubt that patulin was an effective treatment for the common cold. However, as an added precaution, a second trial was set up, this time under the supervision of army doctors. This time, the results proved to be frustratingly disappointing, and to settle the question of patulin's effectiveness a further trial was begun. Set up in 1944, this trial involved 1,500 postal workers and 90,000 factory workers in centres throughout the UK. This trial proved all too conclusive – patulin had no curative effect whatsoever on the common cold!

Patulin refused to die yet. It was hailed as an effective antifungal agent, then as a possible cure for cancer. However, patulin's death knell was sounded when W. A. Boom showed that it was far too toxic to be administered intravenously. Later studies were even to show that patulin was a carcinogen. The reaction of the 'volunteers' who participated in the patulin trials when they heard this news can be readily imagined!

Patulin was one of many failures of the antibiotic age. For each successful antibiotic which entered medical practice there were literally hundreds of promising compounds which fell by the wayside. The dogged pursuit of a clinical use for patulin can be viewed either as an heroic attempt to find a new curative agent, or as a last-ditch attempt to join the antibiotic goldrush, the excitement of which was soon to fade, leaving would-be antibiotic pioneers with nothing but a long, hard haul.

10

Lives of the Four Major Antibiotic Pioneers

History without reference to the personalities of the subjects involved can be a dry subject, particularly in the case of the history of science, which is often related as if scientists work in some kind of emotional vacuum and lack all interest in life outside their work. This approach reaches its extremes in the portrayal of the 'mad scientist' of popular culture, or the image of the scientist as an individual tirelessly working for the betterment of mankind. It is of course unnecessary to say that scientists are in the main quite ordinary people, who take a normal interest in activities outside their work. Their relationships with their fellow scientists are guided by the same emotions as other people in their reaction to colleagues in other walks of life, and often their day-to-day work is characterized by the same petty jealousies or the cut-throat need to succeed which is found in the non-scientific world. Of course, many scientists do have an over-riding desire to help mankind, for example to find a cure for some fatal diseases, or develop methods to help feed the people of the Third World. However, perhaps the strongest motivating force in a scientist's make-up is the desire to find out about how the world works. This desire becomes almost 'pathological' in some people so that they devote their whole lives to their scientific investigations, striving like people possessed until they find the answer to the problem which concerns them. Most scientists, however, can temper this urge to know, and live full lives outside their scientific work. Many eminent scientists are also gifted in other fields such as music, while others have made impressive second careers as writers or even media personalities. In this chapter we will look at the lives of the four principal antibiotic pioneers, Alexander Fleming, Howard Florey, Ernst Chain and Selman Waksman, to try and delve beyond the popular mythology with which they are associated, and hopefully achieve a better understanding of what motivated them in their work. The choice of these four is of interest beyond the obvious fact that they made *the* major contributions to the development of antibiotics. They represent giants in four different areas of science and are also men of widely contrasting origins and characters.

Fleming was born in 1881. By the time he came to discover penicillin he was, by the then current life expectancy, a relatively old man, as Gladys Hobby has pointed out in her book, *Penicillin: meeting the challenge*. The anticipated average lifespan of a person born in 1920 was, amazingly, only 54, and somewhat less for a person born before the turn of the century. Fleming, 47 in 1928 when he came across the penicillin phenomenon, and nearly 60 when Florey and Chain's work appeared, was therefore, respectively, close to and well beyond his assumed lifespan. His major discovery and the fame which it eventually brought came late in life. Yet, as we have already seen, Fleming's name would have been remembered even had he not discovered penicillin. True, he would not have become a Nobel Laureate, and perhaps would have continued to struggle to be elected a Fellow of the Royal Society. However, while his peers did not perceive his full greatness, later generations would recognize the importance of his work, both in relation to his discovery of lysozyme as well as a number of other, less important contributions to medical bacteriology.

Born on a farm in Ayrshire, Fleming followed one of his brothers into medicine, entering St Mary's Medical School in London in 1901. Many fanciful accounts of his youth have been written. I well remember being fascinated as a boy on reading how he would lie beside a lowland stream and patiently tickle trout, until he lured them to their capture. It was difficult for me to understand why Fleming would wish to exchange the peace and beauty of his native Ayrshire for the bustle and grime of London. Fleming, however, seems to have been excited by the move and he soon began to enjoy the pace and variety offered by the pre-Great War capital in its heyday.

Fleming's career as a medical student was eminently successful, earning him a collection of University Prizes. In 1906, he passed his final examination with consummate ease and was then qualified as a doctor, with the letters MRCS and LRCP after his name. He was faced with a number of possibilities in relation to the career he might pursue. However, when Almroth Wright offered him the post of junior assistant in the Inoculation Department he accepted, apparently though without any obvious signs of enthusiasm.

In 1909, Fleming further demonstrated his academic prowess when he again passed an examination with ease, this time for the Fellowship of the Royal College of Surgeons. The possession of the FRCS meant that he could have established himself as a surgeon. In the event, scientific studies continued to hold his attention and he remained with Wright, and he became known as the only FRCS never to have done an operation!

One of Fleming's earliest scientific interests was in the development of vaccines to treat the unsightly and disfiguring skin disease, acne. The product which he developed appeared to work well, and Fleming published a paper on the subject in the *Lancet* in 1909. This, however, was not his first contribution to the scientific literature, since in the previous year he had written two papers on what was called the 'opsonic index'. This test of a person's degree of immunity was developed from the observations made by Almroth, Wright and Fleming that normal phagocytes (white blood corpuscles) were particularly attracted to bacteria which had been coated by something in the blood of people who had previously been infected or vaccinated with that bacterium. This 'something' was referred to as an opsonin and, although apparently present at low concentration in normal blood, it could be increased dramatically by vaccination. Determination of the presence and strength of the opsonins involved the opsonic index, a complex and time-consuming job. Determination of these indices became the key measurement of Wright's vaccination programme, and it occupied Fleming in what turned out to be laborious and largely fruitless work, on which he often worked well into the night.

The introduction of Salvarsan into medical practice gave Fleming the opportunity to further his scientific career as well as set up a lucrative sideline. Since he was well known for the deftness with which he could give injections and remove blood from patients, he was soon in great demand, attracting syphilis sufferers from all over London to his flourishing private practice.

At around this time, Fleming joined the Chelsea Arts Club, where he seems to have impressed all he met with his easy-going personality and friendly manner. He also demonstrated that he was far from the archetypal academic, being skilful at billiards and snooker. In fact, he was an avid player at most sorts of games, in which he invariably excelled. He was also a first-rate rifle shot and through his membership of the St Mary's Rifle Team made many useful contacts, including the surgeon Arthur Dixon Wright, with whom, as we have seen, he was later to do tentative experiments on the therapeutic potential of crude penicillin.

Fleming spent the years of the First World War in a military hospital set up in the Casino at Boulogne in France. Here he was shocked by the inadequacy of the available methods for treating the horrific wounds which he saw. The high prevalence of staphylococcal infections and gangrene, in particular, focused his attention on the use of antiseptics to defeat infection. In hindsight it seems that it was here that Fleming developed the 'prepared mind' which was to lead first to lysozyme and then penicillin. Fleming soon realized that the antiseptics then in common use did more harm than good, because, as well as destroying the invading bacteria, they also destroyed the body's defensive white blood corpuscles. Wright and Fleming advocated that wounds should be cleaned, closed and then protected by a sterile dressing, but on no account should antiseptics be applied directly to the wound. These views, not surprisingly, brought them into direct conflict with members of the medical establishment who advocated the wholesale use of antiseptics.

In the middle of the war, two days before Christmas of 1915, Fleming married Sarah (Sally) McElroy, a nurse and the daughter of an Irish farmer. She was to be Fleming's first wife and her death in 1949 left him grief-stricken. She had been his companion and constant support for 34 years and her death seemed to leave him helpless. However, he was to gain a second lease on life when he married a vital Greek woman, Amalia Voreka, who had been one of his students.

Fleming's discovery first of lysozyme and then penicillin has already been covered in some detail. What then of Fleming the man? We have conflicting accounts of Fleming's personality. He is often portrayed as a shy and retiring man who was incapable of giving a decent lecture and totally unable to engender enthusiasm for his penicillin work. On the other hand, we see Fleming as the outgoing member of the St Mary's Rifle Team and Chelsea Arts Club, who was keen on socializing and always good for a long chat about almost anything. There is no doubt that Fleming generally gave the impression of being a dour Scot and his manner could often appear disinterested. There is a famous film clip in the BBC archive which shows him being interviewed about his famous discovery by Dr Charles Fletcher, who asks Fleming if his contaminant was the same as that which a housewife might find in a jar of mouldy jam. Apparently, totally bored with the whole affair, Fleming picks up a jar of mouldy jam and laconically says: 'Exactly the same. Here's a good example provided by the BBC. Here is a pot of jam and on the surface, on top of the paper, is a number of moulds – maybe the same mould as I got, maybe not. I don't know.' This unenthusiastic response appears typical of Fleming and is one which is hardly likely to convey to someone the impression that they are in the presence of genius! Dr V. D. Allison, who knew Fleming well over many years, describes his character in the following words:

> Fleming has been described as taciturn and laconic, but he
> was a good listener, quick to grasp the essentials of a discus-
> sion and give the coup de grace to any ill-conceived theory.
> ... He was not a good lecturer, but he had the gift of lucid
> exposition and made up in sincerity what he lacked in
> eloquence. His phenomenal memory and quick mind served
> him well in reading medical journals.'

Much seems to have been made of the fact that Fleming was a very bad
lecturer. C. G. Paine, it will be remembered, was of this opinion, as was
Allison. On the other hand, a number of references were made during the
1940s and 1950s to the fact that Fleming was an excellent public
speaker! Here, for example, is part of a report in *Nature* on a lecture
which Fleming gave to the Annual Meeting of the Science Masters
Association: 'No written account could do justice to a lecture which
combined lucidity with dry humour and conversational intimacy.' It
seems, then, that either Fleming must have gained considerable confidence from the public adoration which he received, allowing him to
make considerable improvements in his lecturing style, or alternatively,
people may have been so in awe of the man that they expected less from
him in this department.

Fleming had many non-scientific interests, including art and
gardening. He also had one obvious bad habit and that was his chain-
smoking. Any casual film clip or photograph will inevitably show him
with a cigarette hanging loosely from his lips. He even smoked in the
laboratory when working with pathogenic bacteria, a habit which
would send the modern laboratory safety officer into a fit of uncontrollable rage!

What of Fleming the scientist? A great deal of hyperbole has been
written about Fleming the genius. On the other hand, in a recent edition
of the BBC's science programme, *Horizon*, Ronald Hare went to the
other extreme by describing him as being second-rate. In his recent
biography of Fleming, Gwyn MacFarlane has also made great issue of
the fact that Fleming was not elected as a Fellow of the Royal Society by
his peers until after penicillin had been purified and introduced into
medicine. However, anyone who is familiar with the routes by which
one can succeed to this august body need not place too much emphasis
on the fact that Fleming failed to be elected as a Fellow! Fleming, then,
has been the focus of much misplaced hero worship, while more recent
attempts to redress the balance have bordered on mild character
assassination. There is no doubt that he was not a scientific genius on
the scale of a Newton or an Einstein, but what he did he did well, and
for one of his two major discoveries, penicillin, he deserved all the

accolades that were eventually showered upon him. Fleming died on 11 March 1955. His ashes were interred in the crypt of St Paul's Cathedral, where his memorial lies close to those of Nelson and Wren.

Howard Florey was of a completely different character to Fleming. Australian by birth, he retained much of the independence and rugged-ness typical of colonials of his day. He retained a strong affection for his birthplace, yet chose to work in Oxford, where he was eventually to end his days. He was a first-generation Australian, whose parents had in fact originated from Oxfordshire. Born in Adelaide, the capital of South Australia, on 24 September 1898, he was christened Howard Walter. In 1916, he entered Adelaide University where he studied medicine. Apparently he was not impressed by the medical education he received here. In August 1920, he applied for a prestigious Rhodes Scholarship to Oxford and in December of that year received news that his applica-tion had been successful. The results of his final examination were to fall far below his expectations and, unlike Fleming, his student career was not to be adorned with University prizes. In order to gain a free trip to Britain to take up his Fellowship, Florey worked his passage as a ship's doctor, leaving Port Adelaide for Hull aboard the SS Otira on 11 December 1921.

As Florey travelled from the bleak coastal town of Hull to London, snow, the first he had ever seen, began to fall, and he recorded how depressed and homesick he felt. Nevertheless he quickly warmed to the academic life of Oxford, and soon settled down to life in Magdalen College. Here he made lots of friends and began to impress people with his academic promise. On completion of his studies, he was offered the post of Demonstrator in the Department of Physiology, headed by Sir Charles Sherrington. While working here on certain aspects of neuro-physiology, Florey successfully applied for a Lucas Walker Scholarship at Cambridge, but before he took up the position his wanderlust again got the better of him and he joined a University expedition to Spitsbergen.

Once at Cambridge, Florey again soon found himself amongst friends, and as usual he showed his prowess at ball games, particularly tennis and, in winter, hockey. After a short spell in the US, he was appointed as a Lecturer in Special Pathology at Cambridge. In the meantime, in 1925, he had married an Australian girl, Ethel, with whom he had maintained a long postal courtship. The move to the Lectureship at Cambridge brought Florey and his new wife material gains, based on a starting salary of £900 per annum, which was by no means inconsiderable in 1927.

Florey seems to have been somewhat impatient when it came to

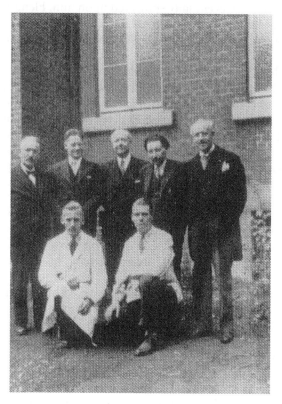

Plate 14 Pioneers of the 'antibiotic age'. Waksman is standing on the extreme left, next to Howard Florey. Chain is standing in the back row, second from the right. (© Special Collections and Archives, Rutgers University Libraries)

research and was generally known to be a hard taskmaster. Nevertheless, while at Cambridge, he formed a fruitful relationship with a technician called James Kent which was to last some 40 years, including the penicillin period.

Then, in 1932, Florey made a decision which at the time seemed very odd – he accepted the Chair of Pathology at Sheffield University. By now Florey had become one of the leading lights of British pathology, and had the pick of almost any Chair which became vacant in the subject. Sheffield's medical school was then small and ill-equipped, and did not have a particularly illustrious reputation. Nevertheless, Florey confounded his friends and accepted the post, arriving in Sheffield in March 1932. As soon as he became settled in Sheffield, the Chair of Pathology at Guy's Hospital became vacant, and he decided that the opportunity was too good to miss. The response from Sheffield to his successful application was to offer him the same salary as that offered by the London teaching hospital, a princely £1200! Although he decided to stay, it was nevertheless clear that he would eventually be attracted away from the provincial University of Sheffield to a more prestigious post. He was not to have long to wait, since in 1934, the Professor of Pathology at Oxford, George Drayer, suddenly died. A Chair at Oxford had long been Florey's dream, and when the opportunity arose, he did not hesitate to accept the offer and leave the industrial North for Oxford.

The move to the Sir William Dunn School of Pathology at Oxford gave Florey facilities which were unsurpassed anywhere, and with an enthusiastic and dedicated professor now in charge there was little doubt that the School would soon attain the position which was always expected of it. Florey gathered around him at Oxford much new talent. He brought with him his technician, Kent, and was later to appoint Chain who would move on from lysozyme to the work on penicillin.

What then of Florey's personality? There is no doubt that Florey's scientific work was characterized by hard work, devotion and meticulous attention to detail. In these respects he differed somewhat from Fleming, who, in later life at least, took a more cavalier approach to his work. While Florey's studies were both thorough and sound they perhaps lacked a certain flair. One would imagine that had Florey first observed the penicillin effect he might have regarded it as typical of a well-known phenomenon and paid it little attention. For one thing, he was not a medical bacteriologist like Fleming, and would have little of the technique necessary to isolate and study the penicillin-producing mould. Nevertheless, one of Florey's major talents was to become invaluable in regard to the work which eventually led to the purification of penicillin. This was his almost uncanny ability to choose the best person for a job, and to organize team work to the best possible effect. Again he differed here from Fleming, who never worked in what might be regarded as a team. Florey seemed to have boundless energy. He was often as taut as a coiled spring, and unfortunately had the habit of bottling up his emotions and concealing them even from his friends. He would rarely seem to be excited, although, as we have seen, the early penicillin work did prove that he was capable of this emotion. No doubt this front disguised a very sensitive man, whom we know, for example, was much hurt by the fact that his team failed to receive their fair share of public acclaim for their penicillin work. It is not true, however, to say that Florey could not relax and enjoy himself in company. He was, for example, a popular member of the Lincoln College Common Room.

In 1967, Florey married Margaret Jennings with whom he had

worked at Oxford. Their marriage was to be brief, however. He died on 21 February 1968.

Florey was above all else a realist. His gift to the world was penicillin, which resulted from his dogged determination to see a job through. He knew from early on that he was on to a winner, and with courage, vision and leadership he built up a team which together had the expertise to bring penicillin from an obscure culture filtrate to the wonder drug of popular imagination.

Looking back, in 1968, on the somewhat turbulent episodes of his scientific career, Ernst Chain wrote: 'I only regret I shall not have another twenty five years to benefit from lessons in human behaviour I have learned the hard way.' The life of our third antibiotic pioneer was to be characterized by conflict and controversy. In many ways, Chain was to be always at odds with the scientific establishment of his adopted country. In the end both achieved an uneasy equilibrium, but there is no doubt that Chain made many enemies throughout his career. To a large extent this was the result of his quixotic nature, but there were many occasions when, unused to the inertia of British academic life, he had good cause to complain. Chain, like Waksman, whose life we will look at next, was forced to leave his native country in the face of anti-Semitic pressures. He was born in Berlin on 19 June 1906, to a Russian-born father and a German mother, both of whom were Jewish. From very early on he showed prodigious talents, particularly in music. His D Phil. was obtained from the Frienlich-Willhelm University in 1928, for a study of the optical properties of enzymes. During these studies he came into contact with many famous German scientists, including Max Planck and Ottow Warburg. Chain was not only Jewish and partly Russian, but also had left-wing views. Hitler's Germany was therefore no place for him and he decided to emigrate to Britain, arriving in Harwich on 2 April 1933. As we have already noted, Chain regarded Britain as something of a staging post, expecting ultimately to move on to Canada or Australia. By 1933, however, he was working for his PhD in Gowland Hopkins's laboratory in Cambridge. Interestingly, Hans Krebs, who later won the Nobel Prize for his work on the citric acid cycle and who knew Chain at that time, was of the opinion that, at this point in his career, Chain would have made a better musician than scientist. Nevertheless, science held his attention and at the age of 29, he moved on from Cambridge to work with Florey at Oxford. He immediately seems to have irritated people there by demanding that the laboratory which he was allocated should be adequately equipped before he started work. In Britain in those days it was accepted that a scientist would make do and work whatever the shortcomings of lack of equipment (unfortunately little has changed!). We have already seen that Chain was appointed by Florey largely because of his experience in biochemistry, then regarded as a somewhat specialized subject area of biology. In Chain, Florey found a first-rate scientist, but a young man who was often somewhat prickly to handle!

Chain had a remarkably successful career after he left Florey's laboratory in 1948, the year in which he accepted the post as the director of a research centre in Rome. Here, he initiated work on the carbohydrate metabolism of animals, with special reference to the mode of action of insulin. He also took an interest in ergot alkaloids and in a phytotoxin present in culture filtrates of the fungus *Fusicococcum amygdali*, which causes a wilting disease in almond trees. He also, of course, maintained an interest in penicillin.

By 1961, Chain had been lured back to Britain by Imperial College in London who provided him with some superb fermentation facilities together with the use of a penthouse flat! He did not, however, relinquish his post in Rome until 1964, when he became embroiled in legal controversy over the prosecution of two professors at the research centre for corruption and misappropriation of funds. Chain was even accused by a prosecutor of selling abroad a patent which he did not own. Both professors were fined and sentenced to imprisonment, which fortunately they did not have to serve, and Chain left Italy disgusted with the whole sordid affair.

Chain's days at Imperial were to be ruined by bitter feuds over funding, typified by the fact that in 1967, he signed a joint letter to *The Times*, saying that 'I would never have touched the place if I had known how things would work out.' He eventually retired from the Chair at Imperial at the age of 67 in 1973, but, even then, he was dogged over controversy about who was to succeed him.

Chain, whose life was characterized by ceaseless activity, was the only penicillin pioneer whom I had the privilege to meet, and the manner of our meeting says a great deal about how he seemed to mischievously seek out the controversy which appeared to follow him around. At that time, I had just arrived in Sheffield to take up the post as Lecturer in Microbial Ecology in the Department of Microbiology. Chain was introduced to me by the then Professor, who, like most biochemical microbiologists, did not appear to rate very highly the science of Microbial Ecology, nor its practitioners. Chain must have sensed this, because when he learned of the area of microbiology in which I was working he said, in a thick German accent, 'You know, young man, that is the most important area for the future in microbiology,' and then turning to my Head of Department he said, 'Don't you think so, Professor?' Perhaps Chain really believed this to be true, but I suspect that, as usual, he was expressing a statement which he knew would be controversial. Incidentally, I asked him at that meeting what he thought of Fleming. His reply was, 'Ah Fleming, you know he was a charlatan!' Again from his writing from this period we know that this statement, made in all apparent seriousness at the time, did not reflect his true view of Fleming.

Although Chain never believed that the scientific establishment of his adopted country ever gave him his full share of credit for the penicillin work, he nevertheless seems to have mellowed in later life, until after a period of declining health he died while on holiday in his cottage in County Mayo, Ireland.

Selman Abraham Waksman was another refugee from anti-Semitism, this time of the type common in the reign of the Russian Czars. While not a direct threat to his life, this form of prejudice meant that it was extremely difficult for a Russian Jew to obtain a university education. Eager for self-advancement, the young Waksman decided that his best chance of achieving something in life was to emigrate to the United States. He was born in the small market town of Priluka near Kiev in the steppes of the Ukraine on 22 July 1888. By 1910, he had landed in the US and begun to support himself by working on a cousin's farm in Metuchen, New Jersey. It was probably here that his love of the land and agriculture which he had gained through his youth were reinforced. Waksman, however, was too ambitious to settle for a life as a farm labourer but instead looked to enrol in the nearby Rutgers College of Agriculture. It speaks volumes for the US system that this young man, who because of prejudice was denied a university place in his native land, was so readily accepted by a university in the New World. Waksman worked with the characteristic fervour of an emigrant out to improve his standing in a new community, and by 1916 had obtained his BSc. and Master's degrees. He then decided to move to the West Coast where he read for his Doctorate at Berkeley in the then somewhat unfashionable subject of biochemistry. This was an important time for Waksman, because apart from becoming skilful in the art of biochemistry he became involved in collaboration with industry. Throughout his career Waksman was keen to wed together academic research and industry, an approach which paid dividends when it came to his later work on antibiotics. This work was a long way off, however, but Waksman was fortunate in being offered a number of posts, the most tempting, but least lucrative, being a lectureship at his Alma Mater, Rutgers.

At Rutgers, Waksman devoted his energies to the study of soil microbiology. He was particularly interested in the question of whether fungi actually grow in soils or whether they merely remain dormant as spores. Having concluded to his satisfaction that fungi do grow in soils he then undertook physiological studies to try and determine what transformations they actually performed in the earth. He devoted much time to the problem of cellulose decomposition in soils and to the question of how humus is formed. Early in his career, he worked with the actinomycetes, a neglected group of organisms which were then regarded as fungi. During this work he noticed numerous examples of microbial antagonism, but, like nearly everyone else, he failed to make the connection between this phenomenon and the possibility of using antibiotics in medicine. In 1927, Waksman wrote a huge book of nearly a 1,000 pages devoted to soil microbiology, and on page 641 he states: 'The inhibitory effects of filamentous fungi, especially ascomycetes, on the growth of microorganisms has been commonly observed; this may be due to exhaustion of nutrients or formation of toxic products during growth.' This is practically all he has to say about microbial antagonism in the whole book.

By now, Waksman was rapidly becoming one of the world's leading experts on soil microbiology. His interests were very broad, however, and he branched out into marine microbiology, while maintaining a firm interest in the physiology and industrial application of microorganisms. This work led him to take out patents on the industrial production of fumaric and citric acid. This keenness to become involved with industry from the outset of his career clearly distinguishes Waksman from the other antibiotic pioneers; in fact he could well be regarded as one of the pioneers of biotechnology.

At the beginning of the 1920s, Waksman became involved in a disagreement about the allocation of the credit for some research work which in many ways foreshadowed his quarrels with Schatz. This dispute occurred over the discovery of *Thiobacillus thiooxidans*, the first of the autotrophic sulphur-oxidizing bacteria. This microorganism oxidizes reduced sulphur compounds to sulphate, releasing the ion as sulphuric acid. It has an unusual physiology in that it utilizes carbon dioxide from the air while gaining the energy necessary for growth from the oxidation of sulphur. The dispute over its discovery involved Waksman and another Jewish emigré, J. S. Joffe. Joffe, like Schatz later, claimed that Waksman had stolen an inordinate measure of credit for the discovery. Open warfare broke out between the two, and their distaste for one another became almost legendary on the Rutgers campus.

As well as his scientific work, Waksman was an excellent scholar. He had a good working knowledge of various languages, including French, German and Hebrew, and he was, of course, fluent in Russian and English. This linguistic versatility stood him in good stead throughout

his career, because it gave him access to the European scientific literature which was denied to his less accomplished contemporaries.
Waksman was also a keen historian, both of Jewish culture and
microbiology. He wrote biographies of Winogradsky, Haffkine and
Lipman, and of course wrote numerous accounts of how streptomycin
came to be discovered.

Of Waksman the man, we have conflicting views. To those like
Robert Starkey, who was Waksman's close colleague during most of his
lifetime, Waksman was kind, generous and helpful. We have seen that
he struck up a similar close, fatherly relationship with Schatz in the early
days of the streptomycin work. Many of his postgraduates remember
him in this light. Dr H. Boyd Woodruff, for example, said of him: 'I am
among the limited number of people who could speak of Dr Waksman
as his professor. How fortunate we were to have a teacher who not only
imparted scientific facts with enthusiasm, but one who was a true
gentleman and was earnestly interested in his students.' Others are not
so generous in their praise, seeing Waksman as somewhat self-seeking
and arrogant. There can be little doubt that Waksman was an extremely
hard-working and dedicated scientist. In his amazingly productive life
he authored or co-authored some 500 papers and 28 books. In later life,
he seems to have developed the image of the benevolent Jewish grand-
father. Some, however, remember him for his well-developed ego,
bordering on conceit. Whatever his personal failings, there is no doubt
that Waksman was a great scientist who made major contributions to a
variety of areas of microbiology. It seems to me, however, that his
scientific work other than his contribution to the development of
antibiotics has often been ignored, and it is particularly strange that he
was never honoured in Britain. This probably reflects an obsession
which microbiologists had, at the time he was alive, with intermediary
metabolism, an area in which Waksman showed little interest.

Waksman died on 16 August 1973 at his beloved Woods Hole near
the famous Marine Experimental Station where he had intermittently
worked for many years.

11

An Antibiotic Miscellany

Do Antibiotics Play a Role in Nature?

As we have seen, a wide range of microorganisms produce compounds which can inhibit the growth of their neighbours. It might be confidently assumed, therefore, that antibiotics play an important role in regulating microbial populations in soils and other natural environments. Indeed, much has been written about such interactions and many microbial ecologists have assumed that antibiotic production by bacteria and fungi is an important determinant of environmental dominance. At first sight, this idea seems so obviously sound that it would seem not to require verification. Surely, it can be argued, if microorganisms produce antibiotics in the laboratory then they must also produce them in the environment, where they will confer a competitive advantage on the producer. This view of the role of antibiotics in nature was clearly expressed by the mycologist Charles Thom in the following words:

> *P. notatum* is a cosmopolitan saprophyte – it competes for a living wherever decay processes are found – hence the soil is one of its chief places of activity. Then if one studies the population of a moist soil at ordinary summer temperatures and containing enough plant remains to show as humus, we find microbial population figures to the gram such as 100 to 1000 millions of bacteria, a few hundred thousand to several millions of mold elements, thousands of nematodes and other worm-like organisms, protozoa of numerous types – the whole presenting a competitive environment in which an organism to survive must have a defensive mechanism com-

> parable to a tank in human warfare. *P. notatum* maintains
> itself there – is there any wonder that it has developed a pro-
> tective substance of formidable nature in its battle for life?

Unfortunately things are not quite so simple as Dr Thom suggests!
Firstly, the ability of an organism to produce a metabolic product in
culture does not necessarily relate to any similar ability when the
organism is growing in nature. In the laboratory culture, the fungus or
bacterium is grown in nutrient medium which is rich in carbon, nitrogen
and other growth requirements. Under these conditions it produces a
wide range of compounds which are referred to as 'secondary
metabolites'. The search for antibiotics merely involves isolating
microorganisms and then providing them with optimum conditions for
the production of these secondary metabolites. These are next screened
for their ability to kill pathogens and are then tested for their effectiveness, first on animals and then in humans. Microbial growth in
laboratory culture can, however, be regarded as 'pathological' as far as
the organism is concerned; that is, the conditions it meets are in no way
similar to those found in the environment and it is actually under *stress*
in the laboratory. Natural environments contain relatively small
amounts of nutrients and it has been argued that soil, for example,
contains insufficient nutrients present to allow for continued microbial
growth. Under these circumstances, then, it is unlikely that microorganisms would waste precious nutrient resources on the production
of secondary metabolites. On the other hand, of course, it could be
argued that if these metabolites provide a competitive advantage then
they would be worth 'paying for' in nutrient terms.

Waksman was one of the first to consider the problem of whether or
not antibiotics are produced in soils. However, it has been suggested
that his interest was not purely intellectual. This is because in order to
patent any of the antibiotics discovered at Rutgers it was necessary for
Waksman to demonstrate that something new had in fact been
discovered. If the antibiotic in question is produced in soil then patent
lawyers could argue that it is a natural product and, as a result, is not
patentable. It was therefore clearly in Waksman's interest to promote
the view that antibiotics are not naturally formed in soils, but result
from our ingenuity in isolating and culturing them.

Waksman's views on the role which streptomycin production plays in
the soil are summed up in the following words, published in 1956 in a
paper entitled 'The role of antibiotics in natural processes':

> Streptomycin is produced by certain actinomycetes growing
> in pure culture in highly selected media, rich in proteins and

protein degradation products. A single bacterial cell gaining entrance into such a medium is capable of developing so rapidly that it will completely prevent the growth of the streptomycin-producing organism. Since the soil, at best, contains only traces of the nutrients essential for strepto-mycin production and since the soil contains large numbers of bacteria capable of competing with the actinomycetes for these nutrients, the latter can lead in the soil, at best, only a starvation existence. The presence of hundreds of species and variants of actinomycetes in a single gram of soil renders rather remote the possibility of any one organism gaining prominence. Under these conditions, only traces of streptomycin, if any, can be formed in the soil. Further, since bacteria rapidly develop resistance to streptomycin in its presence, one would expect, if this antibiotic were formed in the soil, to find special strains of streptomycin resistant organisms. This is not the case. Finally, streptomycin as a base is rapidly adsorbed by the soil particles and is thus rendered inactive or is actually destroyed through the activities of streptomycin-decomposing bacteria. All factors thus point to the absolute improbability of streptomycin ever being produced in the soil or even ever playing a part in natural processes.

The evidence which is available to date suggests then that microorganisms do not produce detectable quantities of antibiotics in soils. It is possible, however, that small quantities of these compounds are produced when an organism grows alongside a competitor, perhaps by utilizing the nutrients released when the competing organism is being consumed. It is more likely, however, that antimicrobial compounds are produced by bacteria and fungi during growth on decomposing plant residues, food materials or grains. As we saw in the section devoted to the folklore use of moulds in therapy, the production of mycotoxins is highly favoured by these conditions, and many of these compounds possess antibacterial activity. It is less likely, however, that the antibiotics which have found a place in medicine will be produced under these circumstances.

HOW DO ANTIBIOTICS WORK?

Most antibiotics are bacteriostatic in clinical use, although some may act as bactericides, particularly when administered in large quantities.

The former action inhibits the growth of the pathogen and relies upon the body's immune system to immobilize any remaining bacteria; bactericides, on the other hand, kill bacteria outright. How then do antibiotics actually inhibit or kill pathogens? Chloramphenicol, the tetracyclines and streptomycins and a number of other antibiotics act against bacteria by interfering with their ability to synthesize the proteins essential for their body components. The end result is, of course, suppression of growth, interference with cell multiplication and ultimately death. Unfortunately, these compounds may also interfere with protein biosynthesis in human cells, affecting cells which frequently divide, as is illustrated by the ability of chloramphenicol to inhibit bone-marrow cell replication. Penicillins, on the other hand, are bacteriostats which interfere with the ability of the bacterial cell to form a wall, leading to the inevitable cellular disruption and ultimately death. As a result, penicillin kills only those bacteria which are in the process of building new cell walls, or which are about to divide to form daughter cells. Fortunately, human cells are not surrounded by walls as is the case with bacteria, a fact which explains the marked selectivity of compounds such as penicillin. Other antibiotics, like amphotericin and nystatin, affect the cell membrane rather than the wall of the pathogen causing it to weaken or break, or prevent it from functioning. Less typical is the ability of some antibiotics such as the rifamycins to inhibit the bacterial synthesis of RNA. These compounds inhibit an enzyme called RNA polymerase which carries genetic instructions from the chromosomal DNA to ribosomes, intracellular structures situated outside the nucleus in which occur the vital synthesis of proteins. Fortunately, the enzyme involved in this process in human cells is not similarly inhibited.

ANTIBIOTICS IN THE FIGHT AGAINST CANCER

The first antibiotic to be isolated by Waksman and co-workers at Rutgers was called actinomycin, a red compound isolated from a species of *Streptomyces*. Actinomycin unfortunately proved too toxic for general use as an antibiotic – it was even seriously considered as a rat poison. However, in 1952, 12 years after it was discovered, it was shown that a variant, actinomycin B, could be used in the treatment of a form of cancer called Hodgkin's disease.

The recognition that an antibiotic could cure at least one form of cancer led to a thorough search for other anti-cancer agents amongst established antimicrobial products, as well as newly-isolated compounds. In the forefront of this research was Chester Stock, Chief of the Experimental Chemotherapy Division of the Sloan Kettering Institute in New York. In 1950, Stock published the results of a vast screening programme involving tests on compounds sent to the Sloan Institute from academic and industrial researchers all over the world. The results revealed that of the 33 antibiotics in clinical use which were studied only 5 inhibited the development of the test cancer used while none were useful in treating cancers in patients. The scale of the screening programme involved and the limited returns expected from this kind of work can be gauged by the fact that, of over 1,000 microbial filtrates tested, only 5 showed any promise as serious contenders in the role of antitumour agents.

By 1955, Stock's screening programme had been taken over by the Cancer Chemotherapy National Service Centre, at which point some 2,000 chemicals and countless fermentation products had been screened, a figure which was to reach an astonishing 500,000 chemicals and natural products examined over the following 20 years!

In 1952, actinomycin C was shown to inhibit tumour growth, particularly in patients suffering from lymphatic tumours. Then, in 1953, Waksman's group isolated the D-form of actinomycin. Encouraging results were obtained when actinomycin D (or dactinomycin) was used on children with advanced Wilms' tumour, muscle tumours, Ewing's bone tumour and Hodgkin's disease. Actinomycin D, when used in combination with radiation therapy, has also significantly improved the survival rate of children suffering from Wilms' kidney tumour, with many patients living for eight years or more after diagnosis. Wilms' tumour is found primarily in children below the age of 5, and in the USA alone it is thought to infect some 10,000 children each year. This antibiotic has also helped transform the prognosis of patients suffering from soft tissue sarcomas.

In 1956, Japanese scientists reported that mitomycin, an antibiotic from *Streptomyces caespitosus*, was useful in the treatment of gastro-intestinal tumours. Then, in 1962, aureolic acid isolated from *Streptomyces argillaceus* was also recognized as a potential antitumour agent. Other antibiotics which are useful in cancer treatment include daunorubicin, which is effective with combination therapy in the treatment of leukaemia, and adriamycin, which is probably the most promising antitumour drug yet to appear. Although it is relatively toxic, adriamycin remains of considerable value in the treatment of acute leukaemias, as well as many solid tumours. Finally, in 1962, a glycopeptide called bleomycin A^2 was used in the treatment of cancer of the head and neck; unlike most other antitumour agents bleomycin A^2 does not depress the formation of bone marrow.

In conclusion, while the perfect antitumour agent is still awaited, a number of antibiotics are now available which have markedly improved the prospect of patients suffering from various forms of cancer.

ANTIBIOTICS AGAINST DISEASES CAUSED BY VIRUSES INCLUDING HIV

Many of the most recent problems which have arisen in medicine, including hepatitis B and AIDS, are caused by viruses. Unfortunately we have yet to find a truly effective antiviral agent, although compounds like acylclovir (Zovirax) and AZT are useful in the treatment of herpes and AIDS respectively.

With our increasing knowledge of how viruses replicate, it should soon be possible to develop compounds which can prevent viral replication at specific sites on specific viruses. While several antibiotics interfere with viral replication, they unfortunately also damage host cells. Actinomycin D inhibits DNA-containing but not RNA viruses, but it is too toxic for general clinical use as an antibiotic. Daunomycin, another antibiotic which was referred to above, also inhibits DNA viruses, but unfortunately fails to distinguish between viral and host-cell DNA. It may yet find a use, however, in the treatment of surface viral infections such as those caused by the herpes virus. The antibiotic rifamycin, which is derived from the actinomycete *Nocardia mediterranei*, gives rise to a semi-synthetic compound, rifampicin (or rifampin). This antibiotic has become established as a valuable anti-tuberculosis agent, and also has antiviral activity.

Unfortunately, despite the usefulness of these compounds, we still have not found an antiviral antibiotic or for that matter an antiviral drug which can be guaranteed to cure viral infections. The appearance of AIDS has, however, increased the urgency with which such a compound is being sought, and with a little luck the huge funding programmes involved will pay dividends.

AIDS is not a single disease like, say, tuberculosis, but is a syndrome of infections brought about by the destruction of the patient's immune system by the Human Immunodeficiency Virus (HIV). As a result, people with AIDS can suffer from a wide range of infections, some of which are caused by microorganisms which normally do not function as pathogens. Infections which are typical of the syndrome include *Pneumocystis carinii* pneumonia, tumours (notably Kaposi's sarcoma) and tuberculosis.

Antibiotics have the potential to play two important roles in the treatment of AIDS. Firstly, and at the moment most importantly, antibiotics can be used to cure or alleviate some of the component diseases of the Syndrome. For example, tuberculosis in AIDS sufferers can be treated by a conventional regimen of antibiotics and drugs, such as pyrazinamide, ethambutol, rifampicin and isoniazid. Bacterial pneumonia in AIDS patients can also be treated using conventional antibiotic therapy, while nystatin and ketoconazole can be very helpful in the treatment of opportunist fungal infections, such as thrush, disseminated histoplasmosis, cryptococcosis and aspergillosis. However, despite the fact that many of the manifestations of the Syndrome can be treated, the prognosis for the AIDS sufferer remains grim indeed.

Instead of merely alleviating the symptoms of AIDS, antibiotics may perhaps provide a cure. This possibility was emphasized by some recent work on an antibiotic called fucidic acid. While this compound failed to provide the hoped-for cure for AIDS, research on it illustrates the possibility that antibiotics may help to halt the progress of the virus.

Fucidic acid (or fucidin) was first reported in 1962, by a Danish team led by W. O. Gogtfredsen, since when it has found only a limited use in the treatment of bacterial infections of the eye and skin; it has, however, also been evaluated for use against antibiotic-resistant bacteria and in the treatment of cystic fibrosis.

In late 1987, newspaper reports referring to AIDS described what they called 'a breakthrough, an antibiotic which can apparently halt the disease'. These headlines referred to studies on the use of fucidic acid by a team of British and Danish doctors, the British involvement being led by Dr Angus Dalgleish of the Northwich Park Hospital in London. Dalgleish described how he had used this antibiotic to treat a 48-year old AIDS sufferer who had contracted a variety of infections including tuberculosis. Fucidic acid was added to the patient's regimen of drugs and within two weeks his fever had miraculously disappeared and he put on sufficient weight for him to withstand an operation and then return to work. Two months later, the patient had put on weight and the Syndrome appeared to have been stopped from progressing.

If fucidic acid were effective against AIDS, then it would have a number of advantages over AZT. In contrast to AZT, fucidic acid is cheap to produce, and secondly it can be taken by mouth and without major side effects. However, at the time of writing, it seems that hopes that fucidic acid might provide an effective cure for AIDS have been proved short-lived, since recent tests have shown that it has no effect whatsoever on the AIDS virus. Any positive effects of its use seem to have resulted from its ability to reduce the symptoms of the secondary infections which make up the Syndrome.

A recent book by Jad Adams, *The HIV Myth*, provides some hope that antibiotics may yet play a role in curing AIDS. This somewhat heretical account of the disease challenges the theory that the Syndrome is caused by the Human Immunodeficiency Virus. This view is based on the fact that, while some people who suffer from AIDS do not carry the virus, there are millions of people who do, but who do not present symptoms of the disease. Adams also belongs to a small but growing number of scientists who believe that the HIV virus is simply the wrong structure to cause the disease. Instead, Adams maintains that AIDS is related to syphilis. His theory is based on the fact that AIDS dementia is very similar to neurosyphilis, and that Kaposi's sarcoma is indistinguishable from skin lesions found in syphilis patients. Moreover, Adams suggests that there may be a reservoir of untreated syphilis cases amongst the homosexual community, and that perhaps it is a mutant strain of syphilis which is the cause of AIDS. If this were true then it would offer some hope for the future, since, as we have seen, bacteria are far more readily susceptible to antibiotics than are viruses. Not surprisingly, *The HIV Myth* has been vehemently attacked by AIDS experts, who criticize Adams for numerous elementary errors. Some critics have even suggested that that the book is so flawed that it should not have been published, and at best should now be retracted. We can only await the outcome of this fierce debate. In the meantime, however, most experts remain convinced that the HIV virus is without doubt the culprit behind AIDS.

Fucidic acid is not the only antibiotic which is currently under trial as an anti-AIDS drug. Adriamycin (dioxrubicin), for example, is currently of interest because of its ability to prevent the AIDS virus replicating, at least in the test tube, and also because it appears to be potentially useful in the treatment of Kaposi's sarcoma.

Rifabutin is another compound of interest to AIDS researchers. This drug, a derivative of the antibiotic rifamycin, can inhibit the AIDS virus, and since it can cross the blood–brain barrier, may prove useful in the treatment of AIDS patients with brain damage.

Researchers at the Waksman Institute are actively engaged in studying certain polyene macrolide antifungal antibiotics in relation to their possible use in the treatment of AIDS. Compounds such as AME (amphotericin B methylester ascorbate) are particularly interesting because they interfere with viral replication at concentrations as low as one to ten parts per million.

At the moment, the stark fact remains that AIDS cannot be cured. Drug treatment can currently slow down the progress of the Syndrome, while antibiotics can treat the component diseases which infect the AIDS patient. Since modern medicine cannot, as yet, provide a cure for AIDS, it is perhaps not surprising to find that many AIDS patients are turning to home-based cures, much in the same way that 'homemade penicillin' was used in the early 1940s. One such kitchen sink remedy which is currently in use is a variant of a lipid mixture called AL-721, a compound which is manufactured by the Ethigen Corporation, and which consists of a neutral glyceride, lecithin and phosphatidylethanol-amine mixed in the ratio 7:2:1. This mixture has the ability to reduce the cholesterol content of both cell membranes and the HIV envelope. In early clinical trials, it was found to reduce reverse transcriptase activity. This enzyme, or biological catalyst, allows the virus to incorporate itself into the DNA of the host cell, and so any reduction in its activity is likely to impair the infection process. AL-721 also improves immune function and reduce many of the clinical symptoms of AIDS, all apparently without producing any side effects.

The home-produced variation of this compound consists of $6\frac{1}{3}$ tablespoons of butter, and 5 tablespoons of PC-55 (a commercially available lecithin concentrate) which are dissolved in $\frac{3}{4}$ of a cup of water. The mixture is stirred thoroughly and then poured into an ice cube maker and frozen. This formula, along with a number of variants, has been widely circulated, particularly in the USA, and it is claimed that it leads to dramatic improvements in the overall health of people suffering from AIDS.

Stephen Connor and Sharon Kingman have summed up the current situation regarding AIDS in their book *The Search for the Virus* in the following words: 'Until science has the answer to AIDS the only barrier that the virus will respect is less than a millimetre thick and made of rubber. This thin latex line may be the only way that we have of containing the sexual transmission of AIDS.'

Despite the incalculable number of working hours currently being spent on the evaluation of antibiotics and other drugs, it appears that we will continue to have to rely upon this 'thin latex line of defence' well into the foreseeable future.

ANTIBIOTIC RESISTANCE: A MAJOR SETBACK IN THE USE OF ANTIBIOTICS

'Microbe epidemic claims a hundred lives.' So ran the headline of an article in the *Daily Telegraph* on 2 September 1987. The article then went on to explain how at least 100 patients, in 100 hospitals throughout the UK, are suffering an epidemic of antibiotic-resistant bacteria, 'Methicillin-Resistant Superstaph' (MRSA).

The term 'antibiotic resistance' refers to the ability of certain micro-organisms, principally bacteria, to withstand the effects of an antibiotic which interferes with growth functions or causes cell death. As long ago as 1878, before antibiotics were introduced, Kossiakoff, writing in the *Annals of the Institut Pasteur*, discussed the properties of microbes which allow them to accommodate themselves to antiseptics. Paul Erlich later also noted that certain protozoa could quickly develop resistance to previously toxic arsenic compounds. The ability of micro-organisms to develop a high degree of resistance to toxic compounds is widespread, so it was not surprising that, soon after the first antibiotics appeared, organisms quickly developed resistance to their action. In 1940, Abraham and Chain reported that an enzyme produced by the bacterium *Escherichia coli* inactivated penicillin. This proved to be the earliest report of penicillinase, the first β-lactamase, the production of which allowed many bacteria to survive the antibiotic effects of penicillin. Four years later, W. M. M. Kirby showed the presence of penicillinase in pathogenic staphylococci, making it almost certain that the development of bacterial resistance would, by becoming widespread and clinically significant, severely limit the usefulness of penicillin. Amazingly, bacteria have been isolated from Egyptian mummies which have the ability to produce penicillinase, so it seems that the genes coding for antibiotic resistance was present in bacteria long before penicillin was introduced as an antibiotic. Similarly, scientists at the University of Alberta Hospital in Edmonton recently isolated antibiotic-resistant strains of bacteria of the genus *Clostridium* from the frozen bodies of William Brane and John Hartnell, two members of the Franklin Arctic Expedition of 1845. The 140-year old bacteria isolated from these bodies were found to be resistant to two modern antibiotics, cefoxitin and clindamycin. John Franklin's expedition of 129 men left Britain in search of the fabled Northwest Passage. Tragically, all were to perish within three years of their departure in 1845. One major contributory factor to their deaths seems to have been lead poisoning, which they developed from eating food stored in cans closed with lead seals. It appears that the antibiotic-resistant bacteria found in the guts of the preserved bodies of members of this team acquired their resistance to modern antibiotics by being naturally exposed to them in the past, or alternatively, the gene coding for both antibiotic resistance and to lead may have been located on the same segment of the bacteria's DNA. Thus the ability to resist antibiotics may be merely coincidental and does not necessarily mean that these bacteria were previously exposed to cefoxitin and clinda-mycin.

Infection control experts have estimated that some ten per cent of all patients who leave hospital will have acquired MRSA. The latest outbreak, at the time of writing, appears to be centred on Essex, involving bacteria which seem to have originated in Australia. While resistant to methicillin, these bacteria fortunately remain susceptible to two other antibiotics, rifampicin and vancomycin, so the situation while worrying is not yet critical.

At the end of 1970 reports of MRSA began to appear from all parts of the world. These bacteria proved resistant to at least eight antibiotics. The worst reports came from Australia, where in Melbourne, by 1980, half of the city's 76 hospitals were affected. The prestigious Royal Melbourne Hospital was particularly badly hit, and it was estimated that any patient admitted during the height of the epidemic had a one in six chance of acquiring MRSA. Many cases of routine surgery which would have been quickly dealt with had to wait months because of fears that the patients might acquire antibiotic resistant bacteria while in hospital. The problem appears to have begun in the burns and plastic surgery wards, where deep-seated wounds became infected with MRSA and in some cases both skin and bone grafts failed to take as a result. It seems that the resistant bacteria were then spread around the hospital by a patient with an infected foot. They became established on the floors and furniture, and were spread into the air on skin particles, released when the patients' beds were made. They were also spread by doctors and nurses, who carried the organisms on their skin or up their noses. Any sneeze or sniffle could then send clouds of MRSA into the hospital atmosphere. The problem was particularly acute in intensive care wards, where the bacteria can have a direct route into the patient's blood stream via intravenous drips.

Unfortunately, because they were unable to see the whole picture, doctors often failed to appreciate the full extent of the MRSA problem. It therefore fell to the Head Microbiologist at the Royal Melbourne, Dr Ken Harvey, to try and educate them to the implications. As he pointed out, the appearance of MRSA meant that the only antibiotic which was left for use on patients was vancomycin, a compound which, because of its serious side effects, had been rarely used and, as a result, bacteria had not had the opportunity to develop resistance against it. Since no new anti-staphylococcal antibiotic has appeared since 1964, the development of bacterial resistance to vancomycin would prove tragic. A programme was therefore undertaken at the Royal Melbourne to try once and for all to eradicate MRSA from the wards. In an operation led by Val Humphreys, the hospital's Infection Control Sister, the offending bacteria were traced throughout every part of the hospital. They were even found infecting clean linen in the laundry, a potentially devastating fact since this utility supplied many neighbouring hospitals with their clean linen. As a result, two million Australian dollars had to be spent in disinfecting the laundry.

Now, in order to avoid problems with MRSA, patients awaiting surgery at the Royal Melbourne and neighbouring St Vincent's Hospitals no longer spend time in hospital but are brought directly from their homes the night before their operations. This fact emphasizes how dangerous some of our hospitals have become, since the widespread use of antibiotics has meant that they are now widely dispersed at low concentrations, providing the ideal selective pressures for the rapid development of resistant bacteria.

Every time an antibiotic is used the chances of bacteria developing resistance to it are increased. As a result, the problem of antibiotic resistance can only be reduced by prudent prescribing and by making sure that patients complete their full course of antibiotics, thereby reducing the likelihood of resistant strains of bacteria being selected from out of the natural population. An indication of how antibiotics continue to be misused is given by the statistic that some 60 per cent of US doctors still prescribe antibiotics for colds and other viral infections against which they clearly have no effect.

Antibiotic-resistant bacteria can be carried on clothing, bed sheets, furniture and dust, as well as by infected patients and by some doctors and nurses who unknowingly act as carriers. Particularly acute problems arise if antibiotic-resistant bacteria enter wounds during major surgery. About 1 per cent of all hip replacements, for example, fail due to infection with these bacteria. In order to avoid this problem, modern surgical units are maintained with positive air pressures to prevent the inflow of air containing antibiotic-resistant bacteria. In some cases, complex measures have to be taken to exclude these potential killers. At the Wrightington Centre for hip surgery near Manchester, for example, operations have to be conducted in an inner enclosure which is supplied with sterile air, while the patient's head sticks out at one end. The surgeons operate while wearing clothing reminiscent of a space suit, in which their heads are enclosed in a plastic bubble!

Some recent studies have confirmed that a wide range of bacteria are becoming resistant to an important group of antibiotics called aminoglycosides. Hospitals in the US reported resistance to one of these antibiotics, gentamicin, in 12 to 60 per cent of staphylococcal strains; while in Zaire, gentamicin resistance in *Pseudomonas aeruginosa* has reached a staggering 37 per cent!

While amikacin is often used to replace gentamicin, resistance to this antibiotic is unfortunately becoming increasingly prevalent. In Australia, for example, amikacin resistance amongst one species of bacteria has increased from around 3 per cent of strains isolated in 1983 to 22 per cent of those isolated in 1985! A worrying increase has also occurred in the prevalence of penicillin-resistant meningococci, although it is fortunate that these bacteria continue to be susceptible to erythromycin, tetracycline and chloramphenicol.

Bacterial resistance to penicillins can, to a large extent, be overcome by the use of what are called beta-lactamase inhibitors. It is the enzyme β-lactamase which confers on bacteria the ability to resist the effects of penicillin and other β-lactam antibiotics. Two of the most useful β-lactamase inhibitors are clavulanic acid and sulbactam. Clavulanic acid was first isolated from *Streptomyces clavuligerus* in 1977. It contains a β-lactam ring, and while it is only weakly antibacterial, it is nevertheless a potent inhibitor of staphylococcal and other β-lactamases. Clavulanic acid is now commercially available in combination with amoxicillin (Augmentin) and ticarcillin (Timentin). Sulbactam has a similar range of activity against β-lactamases, but is two to five times less potent. Like clavulanic acid, sulbactam is frequently administered in combination with ampicillin.

The addition of antibiotics to animal feed and their increasing and often indiscriminate use in veterinary medicine is yet another cause for concern. In 1978, the Central Public Health Laboratories in Britain issued a warning against the indiscriminate use of antibiotics in animals, drawing attention to two potentially harmful strains of *Salmonella typhimurium* which are now resistant to several antibiotics in common use. The first type, referred to as type 204, is found in both humans and cattle. It has spread rapidly over the cattle stock of the UK and is resistant to chloramphenicol, streptomycin, tetracyclines and the sulphonamides. The second type, type 195, is resistant to all of these antibiotics plus ampicillin, and neomycin-kanamycin. These resistant strains appear to have been encouraged by the widespread use of antibiotics to control bovine salmonellosis.

The US drug industry has been extremely vocal in arguing that the widespread use of antibiotics in animal feed and medicines does not result in an increase in numbers of antibiotic-resistant bacteria. Some scientists, on the other hand, have argued that the addition of antibiotics to feed may encourage antibiotic resistance amongst bacteria, although many experts consider that this practice is potentially less harmful than is the indiscriminate use of antibiotics in the treatment of animal infections. Despite these warnings, 35 per cent of the swine and 10 per cent of the poultry reared in the US continue to be routinely fed penicillin!

12

Epilogue: Some Recent Developments and Future Prospects

Some six thousand antibiotics have been described to date, and new ones continue to be discovered. Mycologists at Exeter University, for example, recently found that the lowly water mould, *Helicoon richonis*, produces a previously unknown antibiotic called quinaphthin. Active against a range of both Gram-positive and Gram-negative bacteria, this antibiotic is also effective against *Trichomonas vaginalis*, the protozoan which causes vaginitis. However, as is often the case with new antibiotics, quinaphthin is toxic and also appears to be mutagenic i.e. causes a mutation in the cell's hereditary material, DNA. In fact, while it is relatively easy to discover new antibacterial compounds, problems with toxicity mean that only a few ever enter medical use. So of the vast number of antibiotics that are now available, only some 70 are used by doctors, five of which originate from fungi, while the remainder are of actinomycete origin. While new compounds continue to enter the antibiotic armoury they often appear to provide only marginal benefits over already established ones.

Most of the new antibiotics tend to originate as the result of the mass-screening programmes set up by pharmaceutical companies, and, as with other areas of scientific endeavour, it appears that the lone investigator making the romantic discoveries which are the substance of this book is largely a thing of the past. While naturally occurring compounds continue to surface from such screening, there is an increasing tendency for pharmaceutical companies to look at synthetic or semi-synthetic compounds for antibiotic activity, hundreds of variations of which are produced by company chemists. In the future 'designer antibiotics' will probably become increasingly common. These are compounds specifically designed, using prior knowledge of the properties of certain chemical groupings, to be targeted directly to a probable weak point in the cell of the pathogen.

Interest in antibiotics has moved, largely as the result of the disappearance of the lone investigator, from the romantic accounts of their discovery to an increasing emphasis on some of the fascinating ways in which they can be delivered to attack the pathogen. There is also a new awareness of the range of medical uses to which antibiotics can be put.

A good example of how an existing compound can be better targeted towards pathogens is provided by some studies by Dr Stephen Hammond and his colleagues of the Astra pharmaceutical company in Sweden. Hammond's group are developing what they call the 'Trojan Horse' approach to the delivery of antibiotics. Initially, they developed a compound which was able to interfere with the synthesis of a major component of the outer membrane of urinary tract Gram-negative bacteria, leading to their death. There was, however, one drawback – the cells were unable to take up the new compound and as a result were unable to function at the active site on the membrane. The 'Trojan Horse' approach was therefore tried, whereby the active agent was attached to a peptide molecule which the investigators knew the cell could take up. As a result, the bacterium was fooled into ingesting the attached toxic agent which then functioned and brought about its death. On closer examination, it was found that some naturally occurring antibiotics, such as bialaphos, operate in this way. Here the antibacterial component again occurs attached to a peptide molecule, which, as in the synthetic versions, utilizes the cell's own peptide transport system to gain entry into the cell where it can then operate. An added advantage of this approach is that bacteria find it difficult to develop resistance mechanisms to combat such undercover entry of the killing agent.

Another example of the improvements which are being made in antibiotic delivery systems is provided by developments in the delivery of conventional antibiotics used in the treatment of peridodontal disease, that is, bacterial infections of the gums and other structures which support the teeth. In the late eighties the American Alza Corporation have developed a product which should help cure gingivitis. This early stage in peridodontal disease causes gums to become inflamed, making them bleed easily and become even more susceptible to bacterial infection. The gum crevices then become enlarged, with the end result that the teeth become loose and fall out. Antibiotics, when given in the traditional way, tend to be ineffective in treating these infections because of the poor blood supply to the gum region. The new approach to the treatment of this problem involves using a fine thread impregnated with tetracycline which is wrapped around the tooth, close to the gums. Over the ten day treatment period, the thread delivers about 2 milligrams of the antibiotic to each tooth, an amount which to be achieved using normal methods would require the patient to receive an antibiotic dose some 500 to a 1,000 times this amount!

Future developments in antibiotic research are increasingly likely to involve the new science of genetic engineering. Scientists at the John Innes Institute near Norwich, for example, have recently shown that it is possible to transfer part of the package of genes encoding for an antibiotic from one species of *Streptomyces* to another. To their surprise, they found that, when they did this, they produced an entirely new antibiotic which they called mederhodin, a mixture of two other antibiotics, actinorhodin and medermycin. Unfortunately, mederhodin is too toxic to be used medically, but the fact that it can be produced in this way suggests that the use of genetic engineering has great potential when it comes to the future production of novel antibiotics.

An unusual antibiotic from an unusual source was reported in 1987. Called TA after Tel Aviv where its discoverer, Eujene Rosenberg, was working, this antibiotic has unique sticky properties. It is a large, ring-shaped compound which is produced by the bacterium *Mixococcus xanthus*, a member of a previously untried source of antibiotic producers. TA kills some 50 different types of bacteria including both aerobic and anaerobic pathogens, that is, bacteria which, respectively, grow in the presence and absence of oxygen. It has the unusual property of sticking to wherever it is applied, which means that it might be usefully applied to artificial joints, prostheses and catheters.

A class of compounds called quinolones provide a good example of the exciting recent developments in antibiotic research. These compounds are likely to have a major influence in the treatment of disease, particularly in cases where bacteria have developed resistance to more conventional antibiotics. The prototype of these compounds was discovered during the 1960s when scientists were attempting to improve ways of treating malaria. Quinolones work by inhibiting an enzyme called gyrase, which bacteria use to coil their DNA, an essential step in bacterial reproduction. Compounds such as norfloxacin, ciprofloxacin and enoxacin are capable of inhibiting a wide range of bacterial pathogens, as well as proving effective against methicillin-resistant staphylococci.

The last and most recent approach to inhibiting pathogenic bacteria which shows promise for the future relates to the development of inhibitors of enzymes called cysteine proteinases. These enzymes help malignant cells and possibly microorganisms, including viruses, to penetrate normal human tissues. By inhibiting their action it should be possible to prevent this vital stage in progress of a number of diseases. A group of scientists, headed by Lars Bjorck, working at the Universities of Lund in Sweden and Freiburg, West Germany, recently isolated a powerful inhibitor of these enzymes from human extracellular fluids. This was found to inhibit the growth of group A streptococci and could protect mice from an otherwise lethal injection of these bacteria. Although this compound has not yet been tested on humans, work on cysteine proteinase inhibitors may reveal a whole new range of antibiotics. As Japanese workers have found these inhibitors in a variety of soil actinomycetes and fungi, we may yet see a return to a Rutgers-style screening search for organisms which produce variants of these new and potentially useful compounds.

FUTURE PROSPECTS: THE END OF ANTIBIOTICS?

A recent report by the World Health Organization predicted that antibiotics will one day be completely replaced by vaccines. Vaccines against malaria, leprosy and sleeping sickness will transform life in those areas where these diseases are prevelant, while vaccines against respiratory diseases and diarrhoea will be of more general benefit. Dr Kenneth Warren, Director of Health Sciences at the Rockefeller Foundation, foresees the development of a super pox vaccine which could be effective in treating as many as 20 different diseases. By exploiting this approach, antibodies have already been raised against influenza, herpes, and hepatitis B, and it is likely that vaccines against bacteria could similarly be developed. This last possibility has been highlighted by some recent work at the Wellcome Foundation in London, where vaccines have been developed against *Streptococcus mutans*, a bacterium involved in tooth decay.

Yet another approach to combating bacterial infections, which may one day help replace the use of some antibiotics, is what is termed 'bacteriotherapy'. This approach was first attempted during the early years of this century. It involves the use of a living but non-pathogenic strain of bacterium which is used to combat the pathogen involved. Modern bacteriotherapy (often called probiotics) has been used to treat bowel infections, where a patient is given, each day for three days, a glass of milk containing some ten million bacteria belonging to a non-pathogenic strain of *Clostridium*. This non-pathogenic strain then out-competes the pathogen with the result that there is a noticeable decrease in symptoms such as diarrhoea. Another example of the use of this approach to therapy is provided by the use of lactobacilli and species of *Bifidobacterium*, the bacteria found in yoghurt, to treat successfully vaginal thrush and cystitis. It is also claimed that *Bifidobacterium bifidum* and its close relative *B. acidophilus*, both of which are added to various brands of so-called 'live' yoghurt, can aid acid digestion, improve the efficiency of the immune system, guard against internal upsets, and even replace the natural bacterial flora of the body which is removed during antibiotic therapy. Topical application can, like ordinary yoghurt, also be useful in the treatment of thrush and for soothing sunburn; some people even use these *Bifidiobacterium* yoghurts as a skin-toning treatment.

It is likely that in the future genetically modified strains of non-pathogenic microorganisms will be developed to compete against even the most virulent of pathogens, making bacteriotherapy a useful alternative to the use of antibiotics.

It remains probable that in the not too distant future new approaches to the treatment of infectious disease will appear which will gradually begin to replace the use of antibiotics. This revolution in medicine may not be as far away as we might imagine. However, we should perhaps not be too hasty in writing off the antibiotics. Dr F. R. Batchelor of Beecham's Pharmaceuticals has recently commented on their predicted demise as follows: 'I do not believe that the latest headlines signal the end of the antibiotic era any more than did those in the past. Today – 50 years after its first clinical use [sic] – penicillin G is still a valuable and widely used antibiotic and the more recently introduced (but still nearly 20 years old) amoxycilin is the most frequently prescribed drug in Europe and America.' The impact of antibiotics on medicine can perhaps be best appreciated from the fact that in 1920 the life expectancy of the average American was around 54 years, while a baby born today can expect to live until he or she is nearly 75; it has been calculated that ten years of this improvement in life expectancy has resulted directly from the introduction of antibiotics!

Whatever the ultimate fate of antibiotics, there is no doubt we will continue to owe a tremendous debt of gratitude to all those pioneers who laboured tirelessly to make 'the golden age of antibiotics'.

Further Reading

CHAPTER 1

Baldry, P. E., *The Battle Against Bacteria*. Cambridge University Press, 1976.
Lechevalier, H. A., *Three Centuries of Microbiology*. McGraw Hill, New York, 1965.
Reid, R., *Microbes and Men*. BBC Publications, London, 1974.
Sneader, W., *Drug Discovery: the evolution of modern medicines*. John Wiley, Chichester, 1985.
Raper, K., 'A decade of antibiotics in America'. *Mycologia*, 43, 605–774, 1952.
Carter, L., 'Debut of a drug'. *Nursing Mirror*, 155, 21–2, 1982.

CHAPTERS 2–6

Bickel, L., *Rise up to Life*. Angus and Robertson, London, 1972.
Clark, R. W., *The Life of Ernst Chain: penicillin and beyond*. Weidenfeld and Nicholson, London, 1988.
Hare, R., *The Birth of Penicillin and the Disarming of the Microbes*. George Allen and Unwin, London, 1975.
Hare, R., 'New light on the history of penicillin'. *Medical History*, 26, 1–24, 1982.
Hobby, G. L. *Penicillin: meeting the challenge*. Yale University Press, New Haven, 1985.
Liebenau, J., 'The British success with penicillin'. *Social Studies in Science*, 17, 68–86, 1987.
MacFarlane, G., *Alexander Fleming: the man and the myth*. Chatto and Windus, London, 1984.
Masters, D., *Miracle Drug: the inner history of penicillin*. Eyre and Spottis-woode, London, 1946.

Sheenan, J. C., *The Enchanted Ring: the untold story of penicillin*. MIT Press, Boston, 1982.

Wainwright, M., 'The history of the therapeutic use of crude penicillin'. *Medical History*, 31, 41–50, 1987.

Wainwright, M., 'Fleming did discover penicillin'. *Society of General Microbiology Quarterly*, 15, 30–1, 1988.

Wainwright, M. and H. T. Swan, 'C. G. Paine and the earliest surviving records of penicillin therapy'. *Medical History*, 30, 42–56, 1986.

Williams, T. I., *Howard Florey: penicillin and after*. Oxford University Press, 1984.

CHAPTER 7

Coley Nauts, H., 'Bacterial products in the treatment of cancer: past, present and future'. *Bacteria and Cancer*, J. Jeljaszewicz, G. Pulverer and W. Roskowski (eds), Academic Press, London, 1982, pp. 1–25.

Simmons, S. W., 'A bactericidal principle in excretions of surgical maggots which destroys important etiological agents of pyogenic infections'. *Journal of Bacteriology*, 30, 253–67, 1935.

Wainwright, M. 'Maggot therapy – a backwater in the fight against bacterial infection'. *Pharmacy in History*, 30, 19–26, 1988.

Wainwright, M. 'Moulds in ancient and more recent medicine'. *Mycologist*, 3, 21–3, 1989.

Wainwright, M., 'Besredka's antivirus in relation to Fleming's initial views on the nature of penicillin'. *Medical History*, 1990 (in press).

CHAPTER 8

Comroe, J. H., 'Paydirt: the story of streptomycin'. *American Review of Respiratory Disease*, 117, 773–81, 1978.

Epstein, S. and B. Williams, *Miracles from Microbes: the road to streptomycin*. Rutgers University Press, New Brunswick, 1946.

Wainwright, M., 'Selman Abraham Waksman and the streptomycin controversy'. *Society of General Microbiology Quarterly*, 15, 90–2, 1988.

Waksman, S. A., *My Life with the Microbes*. Simon and Schuster, New York, 1954.

Waksman, S. A., *The Conquest of Tuberculosis*. University of California Press, Berkeley, 1965.

CHAPTER 9

Baldwin, R. S., *The Fungus Fighters*. Cornell University Press, Ithaca, 1981.

Bordley, J. and A. M. Harvey, *Two Centuries of American Medicine*. W. B. Saunders, Philadelphia, 1976.

Chambers, S. O. and F. D. Weidman, 'A fungistatic strain of *Bacillus subtilis* isolated from normal toes'. *Archives of Dermatology and Syphilology*, 18, 568–72, 1928.

Finland, M. 'Twenty fifth anniversary of the discovery of aureomycin: the place of tetracyclines in antimicrobial therapy'. *Clinical Pharmacology and Therapeutics*, 15, 3–8, 1974.

Miller, J. A., 'Clinical opportunities for plant and soil fungi'. *Bioscience*, 36, 656–8, 1986.

Rolinson, G. N., 'From Pasteur to penicillin – the history of antibacterial chemotherapy'. *Zentralblatt für Bakteriologie Mikrobiologie und Hygiene* (Series A), 27, 307–15, 1988.

Selwyn, S. 'The discovery of penicillin and cephalosporins'. *Discoveries in Pharmacology*, 3, 283–301, 1986.

Waksman, S. A., *The Antibiotic Era*. Waksman Foundation of Japan, Tokyo, 1975.

Woodruff, H. B. and R. W. Bury, 'The antibiotic explosion'. *Discoveries in Pharmacology*, 3, 303–51, 1986.

CHAPTER 11

Adams, J. A., *The HIV Myth*. Macmillan, London, 1989.

Campbell, C. K. and G. C. White, 'Fungal infection in AIDS patients'. *Mycologist*, 3, 7–10, 1989.

Connor, S. and S. Kingman, *The Search for the Virus: the scientific discovery of AIDS and the quest for a cure*. Penguin Books, London, 1988.

Dagini, R., 'AIDS – the quest for therapy'. *Chemical and Engineering News*, 65, 41–9, 1987.

CHAPTER 12

Brumfitt, W. and J. M. T. Hamilton Miller, 'The changing face of chemotherapy'. *Postgraduate Medical Journal*, 64, 552–8, 1988.

Index